STEP FORWARD!

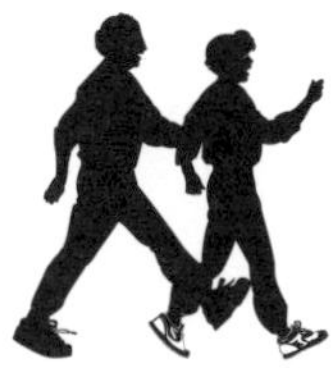

A Christian 12-Step Program to Lose Weight—*and Keep It Off!*

<u>UNIT 3</u>

<u>LEADER'S GUIDE</u>

JULIE MORRIS

Abingdon Press

Step Forward:
A Christian 12-Step Program to Lose Weight—*and Keep It Off!*
Unit 3 Leader's Guide

Julie Morris

ISBN 0-687-08786-4

Note: The Step Forward Twelve Steps are modeled after the Twelve Steps of Alcoholics Anonymous:

1. We admitted that we were powerless over alcohol—that our lives had become unmanageable.
2. Came to believe that a Power greater than ourselves could restore us to sanity.
3. Made a decision to turn our will and our lives over to the care of God as we understood Him.
4. Made a searching and fearless moral inventory of ourselves.
5. Admitted to God, to ourselves, and to another human being the exact nature of our wrongs.
6. We were entirely ready to have God remove all these defects of character.
7. Humbly asked Him to remove our shortcomings.
8. Made a list of all persons we had harmed, and became willing to make amends to them all.
9. Made direct amends to such people wherever possible, except when to do so would injure them or others.
10. Continued to take personal inventory and when we were wrong promptly admitted it.
11. Sought through prayer and meditation to improve our conscious contact with God as we understood Him, praying only for knowledge of His will for us and the power to carry that out.
12. Having had a spiritual awakening as the result of these steps, we tried to carry this message to alcoholics, and to practice these principles in all of our affairs.

Contents

Program Overview—inside front cover
Introduction to Unit 3 4
Step Forward's Twelve Steps 6
Getting Started 7
How to Work Program 9

Session 1: What in the World Are the Diseases of Self? 10

Session 2: Why is Everybody Looking at Me? 14

Session 3: Why Do I Sit on My Pity Pot When It Is So Uncomfortable? 19

Session 4: How Dare You Say I'm Self-Righteous? 24

Session 5: I'm Too Busy! 28

Session 6: Certainly I'm Not Ever Dishonest . . . Am I? 32

Session 7: I'm Scared! 36

Session 8: Summing It Up! 40

Session 9: Why Do I Keep Doing Such Dumb Things? 43

Session 10: Why Should I Change? 46

Session 11: Boy, Do I Feel Humiliated! 51

Session 12: You Mean I'm Gifted? 55

Using Mini-Groups 59
How to Coach 61
Award Sheet (reproducible page) 63
Meeting Announcement (reproducible page) 64
Step Forward Made Easy—inside back cover

Acknowledgments

I would like to express my appreciation to everyone who has helped me with Step Forward over the past six years—especially Claire Bachofer, Sandra Vinson, Dolf Seeds, Marlene Lawley, Dale Heis, Lorrie Greer, Sue Mackle, Rachel Draper, Katherine Coleman, Nicole Barlow, Mimi Adams, Melanie Jones, Shirley Jones, Jean Hunt, Rebecca Pearce, and Bill Hay. I also would like to thank all of the Step Forward leaders and group members for proving that the Step Forward program really works!

I would like to dedicate this work to my precious husband, who has supported me and encouraged me all these years.

INTRODUCTION TO UNIT 3

Welcome to the third unit in Step Forward. In this unit we will complete Step Four and go through Step Seven.

We started our **Fourth Step** (**"Made a searching and fearless moral inventory of ourselves"**) in the last unit. As you recall, we spent three weeks doing an inventory of our past and three weeks looking at the present character defects of false guilt, resentments, and lust.

We continue our Fourth Step in Unit 3 by looking at character defects that have one thing in common: each of them causes us to put "self" in the highest place. As we inventory these "diseases of self," self-consciousness, self-pity, selfishness, and so forth, we recognize how they have contributed to the unmanageability of our lives.

Next we inventory feelings such as fear, poor priorities, and dishonesty. While we are studying what the Bible says about each of these, we begin to learn how to turn from them. It's not hard to inventory weaknesses in our group because we are doing it together. We know when we do our Fourth Step, we don't have to change ourselves. We're just taking inventory.

Step Five (**"Admitted to God, to ourselves, and to another human being the exact nature of our wrongs"**) sounds scary, but it's not. It's a relief to get things out in the open and talk about them with someone who understands. We feel good because we are reminded that when we confess our sins, God forgives us. We are free from guilt, and we feel good because we are in the process of surrendering these areas to God.

I used to think that there wasn't anything to **Step Six** (**"Were entirely ready to have God remove all these defects of character"**). Who wouldn't be ready to have God remove all of our defects? Most of us struggle with this step and don't even know it. To take Step Six, we look at each of our defects of character and decide what they're doing to harm us and what they're doing to "help" us. We must believe that even the worst defects do things to help us, or we wouldn't do them. For example, rage helps Mary to manipulate others because they are afraid she will explode. Fear gives Joe an excuse not to do difficult things. It is only when we realize that our defects are doing more to harm us than to help us that we become ready to have God remove them.

While taking the Sixth Step we take a Temperament Test to see why some defects are harder than others to get rid of. We can stop beating ourselves up for the way we are and become ready to let God change us.

Step Seven (**"Humbly asked him to remove our shortcomings"**) focuses on humility. In order to understand what humility is, we contrast it with humiliation; many Christians get them confused. We are warned in the Bible to stay away from pride, but God tells us that he doesn't want us to be humiliated either. Humble people know "WHOSE" they are and base their self-worth on that.

As we ask God to remove our shortcomings, we learn how to run the RIGHT RACE and not the RAT RACE. When running the right race, we are able to prioritize our actions, thoughts, time, and calories more effectively.

There's no better way to change races and no better time than Step Seven to do it, so we take a Spiritual Gifts Test. This helps us learn what our gifts are and begin to plan ways to use them. As we take Step Seven, we prepare for the miracle of removed shortcomings. The empty space that was filled with too much food, anger, fear, and so forth, is now being filled with good things.

This program is designed so that newcomers may join any time. Be sure that they read the introduction in Unit 1 of the participant's workbook. and get a coach, someone who has been working program since Step 1. A review for leaders of topics such as getting started, how to organize mini-groups, how to work program, and how to coach can be found in the back pages of this leader's guide.

You may contact me at:

Julie Morris
2663 Valleydale Rd.
Suite 266
Birmingham, AL 35244

My email address is:
stpforward@aol.com

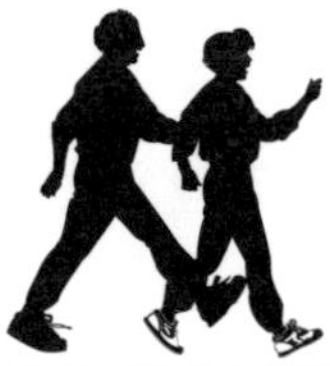

STEP FORWARD'S TWELVE STEPS

Step 1 We admitted that we were powerless over food and that our lives had become unmanageable.

Step 2 Came to believe that God, through Jesus Christ, could restore us to sanity.

Step 3 Made a decision to turn our will and our lives over to the care of God through Jesus Christ.

Step 4 Made a searching and fearless moral inventory of ourselves.

Step 5 Admitted to God, to ourselves, and to another human being the exact nature of our wrongs.

Step 6 Were entirely ready to have God remove all these defects of character.

Step 7 Humbly asked God to remove our shortcomings.

Step 8 Made a list of all persons we have harmed, and became willing to make amends to them all.

Step 9 Made direct amends to such people wherever possible, except when to do so would injure them or others.

Step 10 Continued to take personal inventory and when we were wrong, promptly admitted it.

Step 11 Sought through prayer and meditation to improve our conscious contact with God through Jesus Christ, praying for knowledge of his will for us and for the power to carry that out.

Step 12 Having had a spiritual awakening, tried to carry this message to compulsive overeaters and to practice these principles in all our affairs.

By first recognizing our need for God's help (Step 1) and then focusing on God's ability (Step 2), we come to a point at which we are able to make a decision to surrender our will and every aspect of our lives (including our eating) to God's care (Step 3). Then we learn to recognize and surrender our weaknesses, sins, and broken relationships to God (Steps 4–9). Maintenance steps teach us to continue to walk closely with God on a daily basis, to rely on God's grace, and to share what he is teaching us with others (Steps 10–12).

As we work the Twelve Steps presented in the sessions of the four units, share insights from the Bible relating to the steps, and use the Stepping Stones of the Step Forward program, we learn how to deal with our problems and our feelings rather than eating over them. We learn to cast our cares on the Lord and not the refrigerator.

GETTING STARTED

1. **Who can lead a Step Forward Group?** Anyone with a desire to quit overeating and a desire to know the Lord better. Leader's guides are written in such a way that you don't have to have great biblical knowledge or experience in teaching. If you wish, you can take turns with other members in being the group leader.

2. **How do I find interested people?** Start with a few friends at church or in your neighborhood. For a larger group, ask them to ask their friends. Run a notice in the church bulletin or newsletter and/or in the religion section of the city newspaper. Put posters on bulletin boards in grocery stores, churches, and Christian bookstores.

3. **How do I start?** Read the introduction in the participant's workbook and the first session in both books, pray, and you're ready.

4. **What size should classes be?** Twelve is an ideal size, but groups can range from two to twenty-five.

5. **Can anyone join?** Whether the group is coeducational is up to you. Young teenagers should have their own group, as adults have difficulty being open in the presence of children. Anorexics and bulimics may join, but encourage them to get individual professional counseling as well.

6. **Can newcomers join at any time?** Yes. Encourage those who enter after the unit has begun to read the introduction and to get a coach to help them understand how to work program. Give them a telephone list.

7. **What happens at meetings?** Meetings usually include all or most of the following elements:

OPENING THE SESSION

—Opening Prayer.

—Application Question for everyone to answer (members can always pass), usually taken from the previous week's homework assignment.

—Principles From the Word, reading of Scripture meditations from the previous week's homework, usually done in one of two ways: 1) going around the circle and asking each member to read a meditation on the Scripture that spoke most to her or him, or 2) announcing passages in turn and asking for one or two volunteers to read a meditation on each (leaders should be prepared to speak on any passage not covered).

STEPPING FORWARD

—Stepping Stone Survey, a presentation and/or discussion related to one of the nine Stepping Stones.

—Spiritual Focus, usually a Bible study on a recovery topic related to the step being highlighted.

—Physical Focus, a discussion of food plans, exercise, and any other physical aspects of the program.

CLOSING THE SESSION

—Steps Forward, reporting on weight loss or improvement in some way in working program.

—Practicing the Principles, an explanation of the week's homework assignment.

—Prayer Requests and time to pray over each request.

8. **How long does the program last?** Four twelve-week units are available. The first can be used independently, or you can complete the full program, which can take a year. Order new participant workbooks and repeat the cycle for an ongoing group. Step Forward groups probably should not take off for holidays or during the summer, because both those times are difficult ones for overeaters.

9. **What are my responsibilities as a group leader?** Your biggest responsibility is to work your program with God's help: to lose your weight, to have your quiet times, and to use the Stepping Stones to the best of your ability. You also should:

—**Pray for each group member daily.**

—**Maintain a file on each member,** either in a separate folder or as a section of your prayer notebook. Keep track of prayer requests, problems, and weight loss in order to make your prayers specific.

—**Make occasional encouraging telephone calls to each member.**

—**Make a telephone and address list and keep it up to date.** See that all members have the current list.

—**Plan and lead the sessions.** A few days before class read over the session in both the leader's guide and the participant's workbook and fill in possible answers in the blanks in the participant's workbook.

—**Do all homework assignments** in order to be a good example and to be able to share insights God is giving you.

—**Find an accountability partner.**

—**Facilitate group discussions.** Be prepared to cut off conversation if the group gets off the subject or if someone monopolizes discussion. Also don't allow more than one person to talk at once.

—**Show concern for members** who are in the hospital or who have been sick for several weeks by providing a get-well card for everyone in the group to sign and by making sure that it gets sent.

10. **Are there guidelines for leaders?** Consider the following:

—**Don't give advice** concerning problems. Instead encourage the person with the problem to work program, using the Steps and the Stepping Stones.

—**Ask questions that encourage** persons to think for themselves.

—**Share your own experience** and hope and God's promises.

—**Be a cheerleader, not a policeman.** If someone is not doing well, ask questions such as, "How would the Stepping Stones have helped you deal with this problem in a better way?" Don't criticize mistakes; encourage better choices.

—**Guard against feeling over-responsible for group members.** Your job is to work your program and thus to encourage others to work theirs. You are planting seeds, but only God is responsible for their growth.

—**Be patient.** Frequently remind members to work their program one day at a time. Even if they don't do well, encourage them to keep coming to meetings.

HOW TO WORK PROGRAM

We work the Step Forward program by working the Twelve Steps and using the Stepping Stones.

The Twelve Steps are principles taken from Scripture. They show us how to surrender our lives to the Lord: to turn from our old ways (which often have been ineffective and destructive) to a life of victory in him.

The steps are baby steps to surrendering our lives to God that help us to recognize and admit our weaknesses, mistakes, and sins; to recognize the negative consequences of these behaviors; to draw close to God; and to cooperate with him.

The short forms of the steps help us quickly identify the purpose of each one:

Step 1: I can't!	Step 7: Change me, Lord!
Step 2: God can!	Step 8: Whom have I harmed?
Step 3: I'll let him!	Step 9: I'm sorry!
Step 4: What have I done?	Step 10: How am I doing?
Step 5: I confess!	Step 11: I'm seeking you!
Step 6: I'm ready!	Step 12: I'm practicing and praising you, Lord!

We work the steps in three ways:

- By coming to class and taking careful notes on the principles we discuss.
- By doing the homework assignment each week, referring to class notes.
- By applying the principles of the steps to our circumstances. When our circumstances reflect a topic we are studying, we call this a Lab Course (God giving us opportunities to learn).

We also work the Step Forward program by using the Stepping Stones.

The idea of Stepping Stones came from two Scriptures: Proverbs 4:26, "Make level paths for your feet and take only ways that are firm," and Matthew 7:26, "But everyone who hears these words of mine and does not put them into practice is like a foolish man who built his house on sand." The Stepping Stones are things God tells us to do to make our paths level so that we won't get bogged down in our old ways. The Stepping Stones make our foundation strong in him. Our old foundations were weak because they were infested with things like vicious cycles, resentments, and compulsions. When we use the Stepping Stones, we build our steps on a solid foundation.

STEPPING STONES	Reaching Out
Journaling	Fellowship
Honesty	Accountability
Confidentiality	Scripture
Prayer	Food Plan

As we consider each Stepping Stone, we make small, achievable goals and plan to progress (*step forward*) from there. When we work the program and draw closer to God, we finally experience what the psalmist described: Our souls are satisfied as with the richest of foods. (Psalm 63:5).

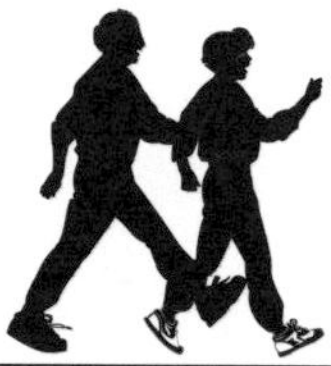

Session 1:

What in the World Are the Diseases of Self?

<u>GUIDING PRINCIPLE: I can make room for God if I get my old "self" out of the way.</u>

Dear Leader:

How are your members doing on their Fourth Step? We are beginning a month-long inventory of the "diseases of self." I believe that nothing can interfere with a Christian's relationship with God more than these diseases. This week we will take a look at all of them, and next week we will emphasize self-consciousness and having feelings of inferiority. The following week we will discuss self-pity and regret. We will conclude our inventory of the diseases of self with a discussion on self-righteousness and pride. I hope you enjoy this series!

OPENING THE SESSION

OPENING PRAYER

Open with a brief prayer asking God to help the members understand that they can make room for God if they get their old "selves" out of the way.

APPLICATION QUESTION

Go around the circle, letting members talk about what makes lust worse in their lives and what they are going to do about it.

PRINCIPLES FROM THE WORD

My meditation for this week is on Numbers 11:4-6 and 18-20, "The rabble with them began to crave other food, and again the Israelites started wailing and said, 'If only we had meat to eat! We remember the fish we ate in Egypt at no cost — also the cucumbers, melons, leeks, onions, and garlic. But now we have lost our appetite; we never see anything but this manna!' [The Lord told Moses] 'Tell the people: "Consecrate yourselves in preparation for tomorrow, when you will eat meat. The Lord heard you when you wailed, 'If only we had meat to eat! We were better off in Egypt!' Now the Lord will give you meat, and you will eat it. You will not eat it for just one day, or two days, or five, ten or twenty days, but for a whole month—until it comes out of your nostrils and you loathe it—because you have rejected the Lord, who is among you, and have wailed before him saying, 'Why did we ever leave Egypt?'"'"

O God, I see myself in these verses so clearly. I used to live just like the Israelites. When I was on a diet, I complained and grumbled. I would long for the good old days when I ate anything I wanted. Like the Israelites, I said that I got all of these things at no cost, refusing to recognize that food was ruining my health and interfering with my emotional and spiritual well-being as well. I was imprisoned by my lust for food, and you were in the process of setting me free, but I complained ungratefully.

After dieting for awhile with this negative attitude, I always would get fed up and begin a frenzy of eating until I was so stuffed that, like the Israelites, I felt that food would come out of my nose. Eventually I got sick of feeling like this and being scared watching myself gain weight so quickly. Soon I would start another diet, and the vicious cycle would start over again.

Over 16 years ago you showed me what recovery was really like. I recognized that you were feeding me with just the foods that I needed. Instead of feeling deprived, you helped me to understand that healthy eating was a gift! Once I admitted that I was powerless over my lust for food and recognized that you could help me, you gave me the power I needed to bring me into your promised land of recovery. Thank you, Lord, that I vividly recall those terrible experiences of being so out of control with my eating; I don't want to go back to that place! Thank you for the manna that you provide for me every day. Thank you that my soul is satisfied as with the richest of foods, and I have learned to rejoice in the wonderful provision you have made for me.

STEPPING FORWARD

STEPPING STONE SURVEY

This is a good time to review the Stepping Stones since we are starting a new section. Ask members to volunteer ways they use each Stepping Stone.

SPIRITUAL FOCUS

This week we will continue our Fourth Step inventory by exploring the diseases of self.

Point out the illustration in the participants' workbook on the diseases of self. After the members fill in the blanks below each picture, talk with them about why they chose each one. (See the answers on the next page.)

Offer the following suggestions if they are not given during the discussion.

- ***Self-centered:*** **self + pride.** The arrows in the cartoon represent that everything comes from the self-centered individual. He is trying to run the world.
- ***Selfish:*** **self + greed.** The grasping arms in the cartoon show that the selfish individual is grabbing everything he can for himself.
- ***Self-absorbed:*** **self + obsession.** The arrows represent that the self-absorbed individual is very introspective and unable (or unwilling) to focus outside of himself.
- ***Self-conscious:*** **self + inferiority.** The arrows represent that the self-conscious individual feels that everyone is looking at him.
- ***Self-pity:*** **self + envy.** The frowny face is self-explanatory!
- ***Self-righteous:*** **self + superiority.** The halo on the self-righteous cartoon tells you how he feels about himself.

Point out that the right relationship with God has a cartoon of the cross of Christ with the individual at the foot of the cross. In each of the other cartoons the cross is at the characters' feet.

Have group members take turns reading the related Scriptures. After each Scripture ask the group as a whole to answer the questions. The results of each one always will include being a poor testimony to others, diminished intimacy with God, and a barrier to recovery.

There are many right answers for each one. I'm just giving you a few.

Self-centered

Results:

- People get angry when I try to control them.
- I get angry when others don't do what I say to do.
- I assume codependent over-responsibility and blame myself when others fail.
- I am playing God in others' lives and this interferes with my relationship with God and others.

The Diseases of Self

Look at the following list of the diseases of self. Decide which picture each disease describes. Write the disease of self below each picture.

• Self- centered	• Self-ish	• Self-pity
• Self-absorbed	• Self- conscious	• Self-righteous

Then decides which one fits the following description:

• Right relationship with God and self

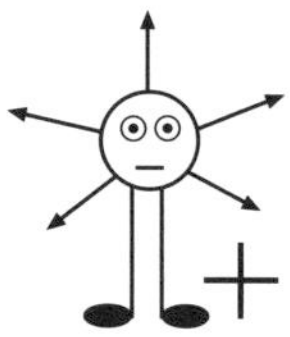

self-centered

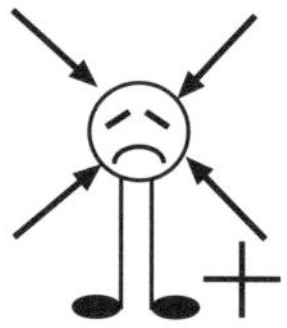

self-conscious

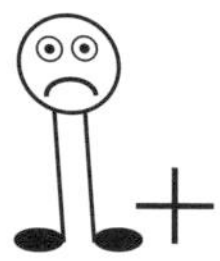

self-pity

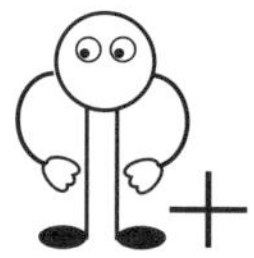

selfish

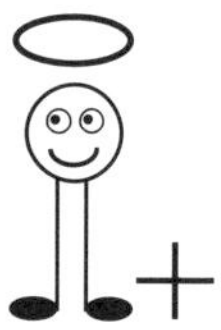

self-righteous

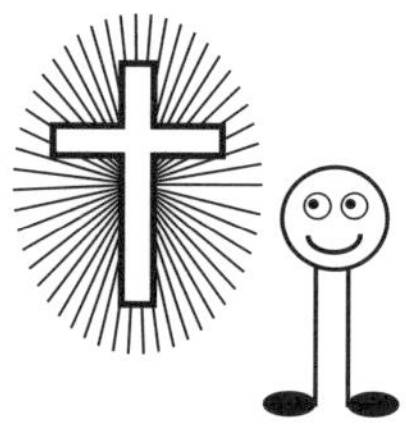

right relationship with God and self

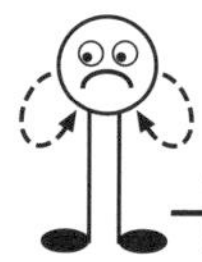

self-absorbed

Selfish

Types:
- Selfish with money.
- Selfish with love.
- Selfish with time.

Results:
- I lose my reward from God in heaven. (I still get to go to heaven if I am a Christian, but I won't have as great a reward.)
- People don't like me. I hurt feelings.
- People won't share with me.
- I lose many of my blessings from God on earth.
- I may become a hoarder, a miser.

Self-absorbed

Types:
- Hypochondria—always worried about every little ache or pain.
- Body image—many people with eating disorders have this. They think about being fat all the time. They may be obsessed with looking good enough, young enough, or thin enough.
- Interests and hobbies—many people can only think about their things or their interests to the exclusion of others.

Results:
- Others feel I don't care about them.
- I am boring.
- People don't like me.
- I may waste my days in unimportant pursuits and become materialistic.
- I may forget about God being there to help me.

Self-conscious

Results:
- I live in fear.
- I miss out on opportunities to minister to others.
- People may misunderstand and think I am not interested in them.
- I get so stuck in shame that my growth is limited.
- When I tear myself down, others lose respect for me.

Self-pity

Results:
- Others don't want to be around me.
- I am miserable.
- I am jealous of others.
- I get angry at God for my circumstances.
- I excuse myself from trying to change.

Self-righteous

Results
- People don't like me.
- People criticize me.
- My growth is limited.
- I don't recognize and confess my sin.
- God gives me "opportunities" to humble me.

How can we begin the the process of healing the diseases of self?

Help the members apply the first four steps to this question.

Step 1: Admit my powerlessness over this.

Step 2: Recognize God's power to change me.

Step 3: Turn my weaknesses over to God.

Step 4: Make an inventory of my diseases of self.

PHYSICAL FOCUS

Be sure that you can share a *step forward* about exercise, weight loss, or progress that you are making in the physical part of your program.

CLOSING THE SESSION

STEPS FORWARD

This was covered in the Physical Focus section.

PRACTICING THE PRINCIPLES

Call attention to the homework assignments under "Practicing the Principles."

PRAYER REQUESTS

Ask for specific needs that can be lifted in prayer this week. Remind members to note everyone's needs in the prayer section of their notebooks. Then pray aloud about these needs as members pray silently.

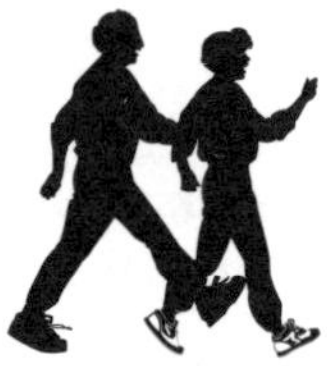

Session 2:

Why Is Everybody Looking at Me?

GUIDING PRINCIPLE: I can be less self-conscious if I am more conscious of God.

Dear Leader,

Be sure to constantly emphasize the first three steps: I can't! God can! I'll let him! If any of your members seem to be discouraged as they uncover character defects, encourage them to call you or their accountability partner to get together for coffee. Sometimes members need to talk about the issue and do a partial Fifth Step (share the Fourth Step with someone). I find self-consciousness (feelings of inferiority) to be such an important trigger in our eating disorders. When we feel good about ourselves because of who (whose) we are, then we will be better able to stand firm against the temptation to punish ourselves by giving in to our cravings and putting on extra pounds.

OPENING THE SESSION

OPENING PRAYER

Open with a brief prayer asking God to help members become less self-conscious and more conscious of God.

APPLICATION QUESTION

Go around the circle letting each member talk about one way he or she is most selfish and what each person can do about it. Encourage members not to repeat an answer already given.

PRINCIPLES FROM THE WORD

Here is my meditation on Mark 12:28-31, "One of the teachers of the law came and heard them debating. Noticing that Jesus had given them a good answer, he asked him, 'Of all the commandments, which is the most important?' 'The most important one,' answered Jesus, 'is this: "Hear, O Israel, the Lord our God, the Lord is one. Love the Lord your God with all your heart and with all your soul and with all your mind and with all your strength." The second is this: "Love your neighbor as yourself." There is no commandment greater than these.'"

Lord, you command me to love you with all of my heart, my emotions. How embarrassed I am sometimes to be emotional over you. When the tears fall at church as we sing praise songs or when a Scripture touches my heart, my eyes immediately want to focus on myself and not on you. I know that Satan is encouraging this self-consciousness, and I ask you to help me to keep looking at you in these times, being unafraid to show my emotions even in front of strangers.

We are commanded to love you with all of our soul, our innermost place where your spirit dwells. Father, help me to love you with all of my soul on a spiritual plane, not trying to understand you from an earthly perspective, just communing with you in oneness of spirit, enjoying you, worshiping you.

We are also commanded to love you with all of our mind, our intellect. Help me to be disciplined in studying your Word, learning your precepts. Help me to memorize them and research their context, their cultural foundation, and their historical significance. Help me to use my mind to love you, not just relying on my emotions and my spirit.

And help me to love you with all of my strength, my actions. I notice that this comes last, as a result of the first three types of love. Only when I love you with my heart, soul, and mind are my resulting good works pleasing to you. So many times I do good works to impress you and others, rather than because I love you so much that I want to demonstrate that love to you. Help me, Lord, to love you with all of my strength.

Your second command, "Love your neighbor as yourself," is really two commands. The implied command is that we love ourselves. The eating disordered can do hateful things to their bodies, starving them, bloating them, going from one extreme to the other, filling them with fats and sugars until they feel that they will burst. Oh God, help me to love myself and to be good to my body.

Help me to love my neighbors as much as I love myself. Sometimes that's the trouble; I don't like myself, and that negativity spreads to everyone around me. Lord, help me to love myself and my neighbors.

I praise you for making your commands so specific and clear. Help me as I do my inventory to recognize the areas in which I fall short.

STEPPING FORWARD

STEPPING STONE SURVEY

What happens if I don't use all of the Stepping Stones when I am walking over unsteady territory?

Use the analogy of walking over a muddy creek bed with stepping stones placed carefully across it. Provide the answers below as needed.

- I may fall and get hurt.
- I may get stuck in the mud and quit progressing.
- I make my journey harder on myself and have to make leaps, rather than walking comfortably.
- I slip frequently.
- I get weighted down with yucky mud and feel awful.

Where do I go from here?

Let the members take turns reading these out loud. **Encourage members to circle ways they want to step forward.**

SPIRITUAL FOCUS

This session's Spiritual Focus centers on one of the diseases of self: self-consciousness. **Encourage discussion on the following questions and answers.**

What are the reasons for being self-conscious and having feelings of inferiority?

- Real or imagined deficits in appearance.
- Real or imagined deficits in intellect.
- Real or imagined deficits in possessions.
- Real or imagined deficits in actions or accomplishments.

What are the effects of self-consciousness?

- Inferiority feelings.
- Envy.
- Isolation.
- Eyes on self and not on God.
- Over-reacting, acting like a know-it-all, defensiveness.

What is the desired characteristic in the place of self-consciousness?

The desired characteristic is confidence in Christ in you!

What is the opposite extreme of self-consciousness?

The opposite extreme (remember, extremes are always negative) is not caring about what others think about you or not taking care of your appearance.

Does self-consciousness encourage humility? Why?

Self-consciousness does not encourage humility. The self-conscious person feels inferior, and inferiority does not lead to humility, but often to defensiveness and acting superior to cover up real feelings of humiliation.

How can I start the process of being confident of Christ in me?

To answer this question, lead the group in taking a look at Psalm 139. Have a group member read each section of the Scripture before each discussion.

VERSES 1–4
Title: God Knows Me
Quality of God: Omniscience

How does this apply to my life?

- What God knows about me: My actions, my thoughts, my location, and my words.
- There is nothing that God doesn't know about me.
- God cares about every tiny detail about me.
- God has seen every terrible thing I have done and loves me anyway. He forgives me when I confess my sins.

VERSES 5–12
Title: God is With Me
Quality of God: Omnipresence

How does this apply to my life?

- God is so near to me, he is touching me.
- I might have trouble believing that God's always with me. I might think about trying to hide from God.
- Why? It is very hard for my human mind to comprehend such an unlimited God. I might think that God is "too busy" to be with me all the time. I also might want to get away a little so I can be disobedient more easily.
- His hand does three things: His hand is on me; his hand guides me; and his hand holds me.
- This indicates the following:
  His hand is on me = He chose me, is close to me, cares about me, is actively involved in my life.
  His hand guides me = He guides and directs me.
  His hand holds me = He holds me, protects me, keeps wooing me to him.
- Nothing can limit God's knowledge and abilities, so I don't have to be afraid of the (emotional, spiritual, or physical) darkness.
- When the worst thing that happened to me occurred, God was right there with me, loving, caring, and empathizing with me. He was protecting me from more than I could bear and planning to use the terrible experience for good.
- God did care. Somehow he has plans to use the pain and understanding experienced as a result of that terrible time. God cared when Jesus was crucified but had great things in mind as he watched his son die.

VERSES 13–16
Title: God Created Me
Quality of God: Sovereign Creator

How does this apply to my life?

- I am to have the attitude of praise and thanksgiving.
- I am made "fearfully" because I am in awe of God when I think about how delicately all my parts are put together.
- The implications of the last verse are that God has plans for my life. I can worry and stew about my days, but I would be wiser to rest in God's sufficiency because he's got it all worked out.

VERSES 17–18

Title: God Is Precious
Quality of God: He is incomprehensible

How does this apply to my life?

- God makes many of his thoughts known to me (through his Word, other believers, and directly). Because I love him, I love his thoughts. I get exhausted just thinking about them all. It's mind-boggling!
- A good cure for insomnia is meditating on God's thoughts (his Word).

VERSES 19–24

Title: Two Responses to Intimacy With God
Quality of God: Patience

How does this apply to my life?

- I can respond to this intimacy by telling God what to do or by surrendering my life to him and asking for his help.
- I can do someone else's Fourth Step or do my own.
- Search me! Test me! (I'm asking for Lab Courses!) Lead me!

How can an understanding of Psalm 139 enable me to begin the process of healing from the diseases of self-consciousness and feelings of inferiority?

- I recognize that God already knows everything about me and loves me anyway.
- I realize how very important I am to him and how committed he is to me.
- I learn that he has a plan for my life.
- I understand that he made me special and unique.

PHYSICAL FOCUS

Encourage group discussion about ways to help a loved one lose weight and things you shouldn't do. Offer the following suggestions if they are not given by members.

Ways to help:

- I can keep my mouth shut about someone else's weight and remember how it feels when told what to eat or that I'm gaining weight. I may mention (only once!) that I notice that he or she is having a problem and if that person wants help to let me know. This is especially true if someone is regaining weight that he or she had lost.
- If this person lives with me, I can refuse to have fattening foods around because it is bad for my program.
- I can keep my eyes on my own plate. This is not true if my overweight loved one is one of my young children. I am responsible for giving my children nutritious foods and for providing enjoyable snacks that are low in fat, sugar, and calories. When they make ineffective choices, I will assist them in making better choices, depending on their age and the circumstances.
- I can be creative and make wonderful foods that are not fattening. I can keep my focus off food when showing that person love, such as buying a non-food present. I can take him or her to a movie, not a restaurant, for example.
- I can show unconditional love and acceptance.
- I can let that person see for himself or herself that the program works and not even mention lost pounds.
- I can realize that "little hints" are usually perceived as "little darts," and I can give up control of that person. (Again, if this is a child, I have a certain responsibility, depending on his or her age.)
- I can pray for that person and model my recovery in the Lord. I can thank God that he is God in his or her lives (so I don't have to try to be!).
- I can do the best I can to work program one day at a time.

Things I shouldn't do:

- Nag that person about his or her weight.
- Buy him or her trigger foods that will tempt that person.
- Make excuses for that person when he or she chooses ineffectively.
- Show love by cooking that person's favorite fattening foods or by taking him or her out to eat, saying, "Just this once it won't hurt."
- Always focus on eating when we do fun things together.
- Shame and reject that person.
- Brag about how well I am doing.
- Drop little hints about what that person should be doing.
- Try to fix that person and take responsibility for his or her actions.
- Do half measures in working my own program so he or she thinks that my program doesn't work.

Calorie content

Go over the chart after group members fill in their answers. Refer to **page 74** in the **Unit 2** Participant's Workbook for the answers.

CLOSING THE SESSION

STEPS FORWARD

As time permits, encourage anyone who is eating better or who has lost weight to tell about his or her *step forward*.

PRACTICING THE PRINCIPLES

Call attention to the homework assignments under "Practicing the Principles."

PRAYER REQUESTS

Ask for specific needs that can be lifted in prayer this week. Remind members to note everyone's needs in the prayer section of their notebooks. Then pray aloud about these needs as members pray silently.

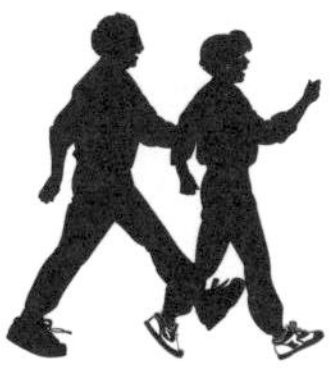

Session 3:

Why Do I Sit on My Pity Pot When It Is So Uncomfortable?

GUIDING PRINCIPLE: I can reject regret and self-pity if I rejoice in the Lord.

Dear Leader,

Are you enjoying studying about the diseases of self? I can identify with so many of them. Each time I go through them, the Lord shows me more and more things that I need to turn over to him. I hope that all of us grow through this series.

OPENING SESSION

OPENING PRAYER

Open with a brief prayer asking God to help members reject regret and self-pity by rejoicing in him.

APPLICATION QUESTION

Go around the circle with this question. Encourage each person to limit his or her discussion to one thing. Some people take great delight in tearing themselves down, so the emphasis should be on the second part of the question.

PRINCIPLES FROM THE WORD

Here is my meditation on Psalm 139:17-18, "How precious to me are your thoughts, O God! How vast is the sum of them! Were I to count them, they would outnumber the grains of sand. When I awake, I am still with you."

> *O God, your thoughts are precious to me. Thank you for writing some of them down so I can know you better. If I focus on myself and become conscious only of my deficiencies, you are left out. But as I focus on you and your thoughts, I marvel at how much you love me just as I am. I am in awe that you consider me as your very own child. My deficiencies fade in the light of your countenance, and my self-consciousness turns to worship of you, my creator, my Lord. You are always with me—beside me even when I am sleeping. Thank you for who you are. Thank you for who I am in you!*

STEPPING FORWARD

STEPPING STONE SURVEY

This session's focus is on Scripture. **Encourage group members to discuss what the following Bible verses say about compulsive overeating.**

John 6:35—Of course, this Scripture does not mean that I literally will never be hungry again! It does mean that when I believe in God (abiding in him, relying on him, being empowered by his spirit), the hunger that never can be satisfied will subside. Many nights I have stood in front of the refrigerator, trying to figure out what I wanted. Now that I am in recovery, I realize that I wasn't hungry physically. Sometimes I was even stuffed with food. I craved something that I couldn't put my finger on . . . and that was intimacy with the Lord and the satisfaction that he brings.

1 Corinthians 6:12–13a—Bingeing is permissible. God won't disown me if I keep on bingeing until he returns! But it is not beneficial. When I am mastered by something, it can destroy me. It's not that God is out to punish me for my addiction, but natural spiritual, emotional, and physical consequences do occur if I continue to do things that are not beneficial for me.

Psalm 106:12–14a—When I believe God's promises (for example, he can help me one day at a time to do anything, even eat right) and sing his praises, I am *stepping forward*. I start to fall backward into relapse when I forget what he has done for me or when I don't wait for his counsel (don't take quiet time, ignore his little nudges, don't read his Word, refuse help from Step Forward friends). Then I'm off to the desert of spiritual dryness and that's when I give in to my craving.

Philippians 3:19—Julie says: *"I never understood what 'their glory is in their shame' meant until I watched one of those talk shows one morning on TV. A large assortment of unhappy, maladjusted people took turns bragging about their misery and misdeeds. Those people glory in their shame (and get paid to do it!), but God speaks about me in this verse too. I was headed for destruction when my god was my stomach and my mind was on earthly things all the time. My blood pressure would have destroyed me if I hadn't lost my weight when I did."*

SPIRITUAL FOCUS

This week we will continue in the series of the diseases of self by discussing self-pity and regret. Contrasting self-pity and regret will help us understand each one better.

Draw a line between each word and its definition:

Self-pity is feeling sorry for yourself.
Regret is being sorry for something in the past, not able to let go of it.

How are they similar?

They both are negative feelings having to do with sorrow. They encourage us to keep our eyes off the Lord and are roadblocks in our recovery program. They both lead to depression. They both occur from a lack of thanksgiving, but both can be healed by thanksgiving when we thank God in and for each of our circumstances.

What is the opposite of self-pity and regret? (Can you think of one word that covers both?)

Contentment is the opposite of both. (There may be other correct answers as well.)

What is the opposite extreme of each? (Remember that extremes are negative.)

- **Self-pity**—someone who has the opposite extreme may deny all grief feelings, keeping up his or her pollyanna mask and pretending that everything is okay when it really isn't.
- **Regret**—someone who has the opposite extreme may refuse to look back at his or her mistakes or painful circumstances and, therefore, will be unable to learn from them.

What phrases indicate each?

You may have to give group members a couple of examples to get them on the right track.

Self-pity	Regret
"Poor me!"	"How could I have . . . ?"
"I feel so bad!"	"If only . . ."
"Why me?"	"I wish I had . . ."
"Life is so unfair."	"How could God . . . ?"

What are the results of self-pity and regret?

No one is more unhappy than one living in self-pity or regret. They are often angry, unteachable, depressed people. They irritate everyone around them and often end up bitter and alone. They can't work program because they use their condition to excuse themselves from the responsibility to make the most of what they have.

SELF-PITY

What is the treatment for self-pity?

The correct order for Steps 1-5 follows:

Step 1: Admit your self-pity and that your life is unmanageable because of it.
Step 2: Recognize that God can help you to be rid of this disease of self.
Step 3: Turn this defect of character over to God and ask him to help you with it.
Step 4: Inventory ways you feel self-pity.
Step 5: Confess it to God and another.

Is self-pity sin? Why?

Julie says: *"I believe that wallowing in self-pity is sin. Look at the following Bible verses to understand why."*

Have the group members read the verses out loud. Lead a discussion on the questions that follow each one.

Philippians 4:11–13

What do I have to learn?
I have to learn that I can do everything through him (Christ), who gives me strength.

How does that help me deal with self-pity?
God can change my heart from one that demands more to one that is content with what he has given me.

1 Thessalonians 5:18

Are my circumstances always God's will for me?
The answer depends on what you mean by God's will. My circumstances are not always in God's perfect will for me. He is sovereign, and nothing happens to me that does not filter through his fingers first. Because he gives me free will, he allows me to turn from his perfect will into his permissive will. The answer to the question will therefore be, "Yes, my circumstances are always in God's permissive will, but not always in his perfect will."

Am I to give thanks in all situations?
I am to give thanks in all situations. I give thanks that God is using everything for my good because I love him and I am called according to his purpose. I also give thanks that he won't leave me or give me more than I can bear. It is not hypocritical because I am not denying my feelings or pretending that I like my circumstances, but I am praising and thanking God in and for them as I am commanded to do.

Julie says: *"Grieving is an important part of recovery. We need to do this when we recognize a loss. A good way to do grief work is to write God a letter and pour your grief on him."*

Point out the homework assignment on self-pity. There is no need to go over these in class as they are self-explanatory.

REGRET

What is the treatment for regret?

The correct order for Steps 1-5 follow:

Step 1: Admit your regret and that your life has become unmanageable because of it.
Step 2: Recognize that God can help you to be rid of this disease of self.
Step 3: Turn your regret over to God and ask him to help you with it.
Step 4: Inventory what you regret.
Step 5: Confess your regret to God and another.

Have the group members read the Bible verses out loud. Lead a discussion on the questions that follow each one.

2 Corinthians 7:10

Does God want me to live in regret?
God does not want me to live in regret.

Is regret a sin?
Regret can be, at times, a sin that shows I don't trust God. Other times it is a result of conviction of the Holy Spirit, so it is not a sin.

After a sin is confessed, is it godly to continue in sorrow to make up for my sin?
Christ's atonement pays for my sin. Nothing I can do adds to his perfect sacrifice. God does not want me to try to atone for my sin by living in regret (but restitution may be in order).

Habakkuk 3:17–19

With what attitude does God want us to replace self-pity and regret?
According to this verse God wants us to replace self-pity and regret with praise and thanksgiving.

What question does God want us to ask?
Not "Why me, Lord?" but, "What would you have me learn?" ***Julie says:*** *"As I am typing these words, I am experiencing a Lab Course in their application. My whole letter to you was lost someplace on my computer, or accidentally erased, so I am having to retype the whole thing. I have a meeting this afternoon with Claire to go over it, so I am hurrying to get it retyped. I could stew and fret over this mistake, but (praise God!) I recognized the Lab Course, and was able to thank God that I had a copy so I didn't have to rewrite the whole letter, just retype it. I thanked him that I had time this morning to do it (even though the laundry will have to go undone!), and I thanked him that I was able to apply the principles that I was writing about and not get upset over this mistake.*

Point out the homework assignment on regret. There is no need to go over this in class.

PHYSICAL FOCUS

Provide members with the following answers to the questions in their workbooks.

1. It has been estimated that 300,000 people die annually in the United States of obesity-related conditions.
2. A pound of fat burns only 2 calories a day at rest.
3. Between 1960–1980 25 percent of U.S. adults were obese (more than 20 percent above a person's desirable weight). Between 1980-1990 this number jumped to 33 percent.
4. Increased servings of fruits and vegetables may decrease the risk of strokes. One study even shows a 50 percent decrease.
5. Exercise protects against heart disease, strokes, high blood pressure, obesity, diabetes, osteoporosis, and colon cancer.
6. Americans spend $40 to 50 billion a year to lose weight, and most who lose it rapidly regain it within a year.
7. People who exercise regularly tend to naturally crave healthier foods.
8. "Light" on the label means that the food has half the fat or one-third the calories of its regular counterpart.
9. Ninety percent of the estimated 8 million people with eating disorders are women. These include binge eaters, as well as those with anorexia nervosa and bulimia nervosa.
10. The number of overweight children has increased by 100 percent over the last 30 years.

CLOSING THE SESSION

STEPS FORWARD

Encourage anyone who has had success in eating healthy or in losing weight to share his or her *step forward* with the group.

PRACTICING THE PRINCIPLES

Point out the homework assignments under "Practicing the Principles" in members' workbooks.

PRAYER REQUESTS

Ask for specific needs that can be lifted in prayer this week. Remind members to note everyone's needs in the prayer section of their notebooks. Then pray aloud about these needs as members pray silently.

Session 4:

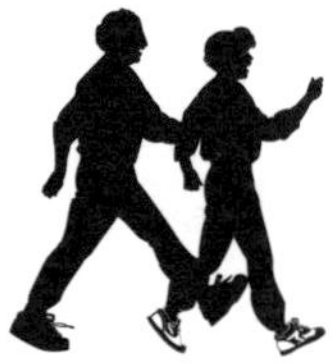

How Dare You Say I'm Self-Righteous!

GUIDING PRINCIPLE: I can turn from pride if I know what it is.

Dear Leader,

This is the final week in our inventory of the diseases of self. We are doing a word study this week. It's good for your members to know how to go to the original Hebrew, Aramaic, and Greek languages to get all of the different meanings of a word that we are studying. This type of study adds such dimension to our understanding, and it's fun too. The easiest way to do this is to buy a Vine's Expository Dictionary. You may also use a Strong's Exhaustive Concordance of the Bible. The number next to each reference refers to the corresponding word in the original language that is found in the back of the book. I am fortunate. I have a full concordance on my computer, so I can research my word origins quickly.

OPENING THE SESSION

OPENING PRAYER

Open with a brief prayer asking God to help members realize what pride is so that they can begin to turn from it.

APPLICATION QUESTION

Go around the circle letting group members talk briefly about the area in which they have the most self-pity or regret. Be sure the emphasis is on working through this issue. You might want to take notes so that you will be able to pray for each person concerning these areas of regret and self-pity.

PRINCIPLES FROM THE WORD

My meditation this week is on Joel 2:25-26, "I will repay you for the years the locusts have eaten—the great locust and the young locust, the other locusts and the locust swarm—my great army that I sent among you. You will have plenty to eat, until you are full, and you will praise the name of the Lord your God, who has worked wonders for you; never again will my people be shamed."

The Lord sends devastation to us. Sometimes he allows us to be defeated to teach us lessons, to encourage us to turn from our sins, and to help us learn how to rely on him.

Locusts may come in any form, but they are always defeating, and if we rely only on the world, they can destroy our lives. A locust may be an unwanted divorce, the death of a loved one, hurricanes, earthquakes, floods, wars, illness, and extra pounds. God promises to restore the years that the locusts have eaten. For some, whole lifetimes must be included in that promise.

Father, thank you for the locusts that you have sent in my life. Though they are never things that I would choose, I can see why you have sent many of them, and I rejoice as you restore me from the devastation they have caused.

How wonderful it is that you

promise me plenty to eat, until I am full! I won't ever have to suffer in constant hunger again as you restore me. I am already experiencing freedom from my food obsession most of the time and know that this freedom will grow even more. I do praise your name, O God, for you have worked wonders for me! I know as I cling to you that I will never again have to suffer shame.

STEPPING FORWARD

STEPPING STONE SURVEY

This week's Stepping Stone focus is on fellowship.

Go around the circle and let members talk about the benefits of fellowship. Encourage them to avoid giving answers that have already been given. Provide the answers below as needed.

- Fellowship with the group keeps me from isolating.
- It helps me to know others have similar problems.
- I am encouraged by others' successes.
- I am challenged by others to do better. (If they can do it, so can I!)
- I study God's Word during my meetings, and it never returns to me void. (God promises that it's never a waste of time!)
- I study the steps and the Stepping Stones and know that recovery is a thing that I can choose one day at a time with the encouragement of my group.

SPIRITUAL FOCUS

During this session we will discuss the final diseases of self in this series: self-righteousness and pride. **Have the members read the definitions of each one out loud.**

What group is a New Testament example of the self-righteous?

The Pharisees.

What did they do that Jesus criticized?

- Did good deeds before others.
- Acted holy on the outside while they were sinful inside.
- Chose the best for themselves.
- Did not see the need for forgiveness.
- Depended on their good works for their salvation.

When is pride a positive thing?

Pride is positive when it means having a sense of one's own dignity or worth because of who he or she is in Christ.

What does the Bible tell us about the negative type of pride?

Your group may recall principles such as the following:

- Jesus rebuked the prideful.
- The one who is least is greatest in God's kingdom.
- We are not to judge others.
- We are to be servants rather than wanting to be served.
- God hates pride. It is sin and separates us from God
- Pride goes before destruction.

Types of Pride

Read the Hebrew, Aramaic, or Greek word and the definition. **Ask for specific illustrations of each type of pride and have the members record these under each word.** If your members can't think of the answers, refer to the end of the lesson, where I have written some questions that inventory each type of pride. There are three questions for each. Read them as you discuss each specific type of pride. The following question numbers refer to the corresponding foreign word. I have written the word phonetically so that you can say it easily. These are just a few of the words that mean "pride" in the Bible.

- **Alazoneia** (al-ad-zon-i'-a), questions 1–3.
- **Tuphoo** (toof-o'-o), questions 4–6.
- **Huperephania** (hoop-er-ay-fan-ee'-ah), questions 7–9.
- **Zuwd** (zood), questions 10–12.
- **Shachats** (shakh'-ats), questions 13–15.

What are the results of self-righteousness and pride?

- Being rude.
- God giving you "opportunities" to learn humility.
- Being a poor witness.
- Hurting others and/or making them angry.
- Not receiving God's full blessings.
- Having a barrier to experiencing God, alienated from him.
- Having an unteachable spirit, not learning from mistakes.
- Not realizing sin, thereby continuing to live in it.

What is the opposite of self-righteousness and pride?

The opposite of self-righteousness and pride is relying on Christ for forgiveness, identity, direction, and power.

What is the opposite extreme of self-righteousness and pride? (Remember, extremes are negative!)

The opposite extreme of self-righteousness and pride is humiliation—the attitude that if I can't be the very best, I'll be the worst.

Apply Steps 1–5 to learn how you can turn from pride.

Step 1: I am powerless over the pride I feel, and if I continue to live in it, my life will become unmanageable.

Step 2: God can help me to be less prideful.

Step 3: I am making a decision to turn my pride over to him and to rely on him to help me be proud only of what he is doing in me.

Step 4: I will inventory my prideful issues.

Step 5: I will confess my pride to God and to another.

PHYSICAL FOCUS

Let the group take turns giving effective and ineffective ways to eat that begin with the letters in the word *pleasant*. Provide the answers below as needed.

Effective

P: Prayerful planning.
L: Location at the table.
E: Encouragemen—from the Holy Spirit, Step Forward friends, and the Bible—to keep on track one day at a time.
A: Amount—eating the right quantity of food from each food group in your food plan.
S: Style—good manners.
A: Appearance—attractively served meals
N: Noticing—what you are eating, how it tastes, whether you are full.
T: Time—eating each meal at a certain time each day and taking the time to enjoy each bite.

Ineffective

P: Pleasing others by giving in when they insist that you have a second helping or eat a binge food.
L: Lying to yourself about how much you eat or how unmanageable your life has become because of food.
E: Eating everything on your plate even if you are full.
A: Allowing yourself to believe that food will fix your problems.
S: Skipping meals.
A: Attacking your food, shoveling it in as fast as you can.
N: No time to eat, so you do it on the run.
T: Taking that first compulsive bite.

CLOSING THE SESSION

STEPS FORWARD

Ask for volunteers to say encouraging things about how their program is helping them. Remind members that our aim is not to do everything perfectly. It is to *step forward* a little every day.

PRACTICING THE PRINCIPLES

Point out the homework assignments under "Practicing the Principles" in the workbooks. **Encourage members to work the assignments before the next meeting.**

PRAYER REQUESTS

Ask the members if anyone has specific needs that he or she would like lifted in prayer this week. Remind group members to make a note of everyone's needs in the prayer section of their notebooks. Then pray aloud about these needs as members pray silently.

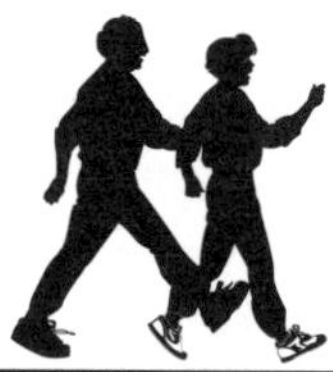

Session 5:

I'm Too Busy!

GUIDING PRINCIPLE: I can use my time wisely if I notice what I'm doing.

Dear Leader,

The way we spend our days seldom reflects what is most important to us. We may spend all of our time and energy at a job we hate just so we can have a few (after taxes, very few!) extra dollars. Or if we are homemakers, we may put more energy into scrubbing and washing than we do into showing our husband and children that we really love them and think that they are special. Some of us may forego quiet times because we are "too busy" and feel guilty when we take time out from our frantic schedules just for ourselves. We become driven to do things that don't amount to anything significant in the long run. Our children are with us such a short time, but when mine were little, I felt like it was going to be forever! I was busier than I would ever be in my life. I wish I could live those years over again. I would have waited to go back to work. I wouldn't have gotten that second degree right then. There would have been time for that when they were older. It's so important that we prioritize our time wisely. As an intensive care nurse I spent lots of final hours with patients, and I listened to them talk about their regrets as they looked back on their lives. So many of them would say how sorry they were that they didn't spend more time having fun with their family or sharing with their loved ones. Fortunately, it's not too late to change our poor priorities! We can't relive our past, but we can learn from our mistakes and can trust God to restore the years the locusts of wrong priorities have eaten. We can inventory our time utilization and recognize ways we want to change.

OPENING THE SESSION

OPENING PRAYER

Open with a brief prayer asking God to help members be more aware of what they are doing so that they can use their time wisely.

APPLICATION QUESTION

Go around the circle with this question. Ask each person to briefly explain his or her answer. Also ask that members not repeat an answer already given, if possible.

PRINCIPLES FROM THE WORD

My meditation for this week is on Matthew 23:27–28, "Woe to you, teachers of the law and pharisees, you hypocrites! You are like whitewashed tombs, which look beautiful on the outside but on the inside are full of dead men's bones and everything unclean. In the same way, on the outside you appear to people as righteous but on the inside you are full of hypocrisy and wickedness."

You warn me here, Lord, to be real with those I teach, not to pretend to eat perfectly or work a perfect program. You encourage me to share my weaknesses and mistakes as well as my victories with those in my groups.

That's hard, Lord! I say to myself that I don't want to be a bad influence on others by admitting to them that my eating was sloppy, I was inconsiderate with my husband, or prideful with a friend. But I guess the truth is that, if I don't tell them the truth, I am like the whitewashed tomb Jesus was talking about. I must turn my back on prideful thoughts that encourage me to wear a mask that says, "I am recovered." I am better, with your help, but I see that I have such a long way to go. Help me to share this honestly with others.

STEPPING FORWARD

STEPPING STONE SURVEY

This week's Stepping Stone focus is on prayer. Have a *step forward* ready to share about how your quiet time has helped you to keep eating right and to draw closer to the Lord.

SPIRITUAL FOCUS

We will continue to study Step 4 by discussing five types of poor priorities. *The Tyranny of the Urgent* (Charles Hummel, Intervarsity Press) is a wonderful little booklet. I highly recommend it!

Poor Priority No. 1: When Urgent Things Overtake Important Things

What are some examples of important tasks?

- Quiet times
- Bible study
- Sharing Jesus
- Using the Stepping Stones

Urgent tasks call for instant actions. What are some examples?

- Work
- Car pool, errands
- Cooking/eating
- Answering the phone

Have the group members take turns reading the following quotes from *The Tyranny of the Urgent.* Lead discussions on the questions that follow each.

"The root of all sin is self-sufficiency." How is this true?
God's will for me is that I rely on him. If I don't consult him for direction, spend time in his Word, praise him, and abide with him, I am sinning. All actions that I do in the flesh (ignoring him) are not acceptable to him.

"The opposite of self-sufficiency is acknowledging the need for God in prayer." How does our program of recovery address this?
All of the steps direct us to a life of prayerful reliance.

"Prayer is like a time out in a football game." Why?

- Time to talk to the Head Coach.
- Time to assess our fumbles and ask how we can do better.
- Time to catch our breath and slow down.

Matthew 6:33: How would you paraphrase it?
Have your quiet time, work your steps (I can't, God can, and I'll let him!), and leave the results to God.

John 17:4: What's unusual about this statement?
He was in the prime of life. There were thousands left to heal, and many did not know him yet. Most people had rejected him and believed he was a fake.

Poor Priority No. 2: Not Saying No

The second type of poor priorities is not saying no — letting good things distract us from our recovery and our primary goals.

Mark 12:30-31: What does each part mean?

Love the Lord with all your heart:

Love the Lord with your emotions.

Love the Lord with all your soul:

Love the Lord with your spirit.

Love the Lord with all your mind:

Love the Lord with your intellect.

Love the Lord with all your strength:

Love the Lord with your actions.

Love your neighbor as yourself:

It is assumed that you love yourself.

What is significant about the order of these?

We put ourselves and our actions first, and God puts them last. If we're too busy doing good deeds to spend quality time with God, we're prioritizing wrong.

How do we know if we should say no?

- If what we are asked to do is not biblical.
- If we have no peace after we prayed about it.
- If we are already overwhelmed because we are too busy; if it will interfere with our quiet times.
- If one in authority over us says we shouldn't do this.
- If our motives for doing it are not right.

Poor Priority No. 3: Procrastination

What are the causes of procrastination?

- Bad habit of responding by doing only what I feel like doing.
- Perfectionism (I can't do it perfectly, so I won't do it at all.)
- Passive aggressive behavior. (I'll show him . . . I won't do what he wants me to.)
- Indecision.
- Fear of failure, fear of pain (rejection, criticism, physical pain).
- Laziness.

Apply Steps 1–5 to help you find the way out of procrastination.

Step 1: Admit that your procrastination is a bad habit that you're powerless over and list specific ways that it is making your life unmanageable.

Step 2: Believe that God can help you to stop procrastinating as you work your Step Forward program one day at a time.

Step 3: Make a decision to turn this problem over to God each day by praying for the willingness and ability to do specific unwanted tasks that day.

Step 4: Inventory areas of procrastination, reasons for it, and ways to turn from it—like making a to-do list and rewarding yourself if you do most of the things on it (not with food, of course!). Another good thing to inventory is projects that need to be done (for example, paint a room, shampoo carpets, wax the car). Make the list of projects as you go from room to room in your house.

Step 5: Admit specific areas of procrastination to God, yourself, and your accountability partner. You may decide to ask your partner to hold you accountable for doing one project each week, as well as other smaller goals, such as writing a letter a week, making Step Forward calls, and so forth.

Poor Priority No. 4: Not Balancing Work and Play

The fourth type of poor priorities is not having good balance between recreation and work.

How can you accomplish more?

Assess what causes you to waste the most time:

- television, reading
- nibbling
- worrying
- daydreaming, sleeping
- shopping
- talking on the phone

Make a Time Management List
A Time Management List is helpful for those who want to accomplish more. Here are some possibilities:

- Quiet time 1 hour
- Exercise 30 minutes
- Fun with kids 1 hour
- Reading Bible 15 minutes
- Memorizing 3 minutes
- Cleaning 1 hour

A time management list is helpful to limit certain activities, for example:

- Shopping 2 hours a week
- Television 1 hour a day
- Phone 1/2 hour a day
- Eating out twice a week

How to Have More Fun
Let members take turns reading the list. Have them mark the ones that appeal to them and add their own.

Poor Priority No. 5: Not Enjoying Each Day

What keeps us from enjoying each day to the fullest?

Have the members talk briefly about the ones they have circled.

PHYSICAL FOCUS

Read over these cooking tips and menu suggestions in class as time permits. **Encourage members to share ways they are cooking right when they are too busy.**

CLOSING THE SESSION

STEPS FORWARD

Invite any members who are seeing progress in *stepping forward* to share their experiences with the group.

PRACTICING THE PRINCIPLES

Point out to members the homework assignments under "Practicing the Principles" in their workbooks. **Encourage members to work the assignments before the next meeting.**

PRAYER REQUESTS

Ask the members if anyone has specific needs that he or she would like lifted in prayer this week. Remind group members to make a note of everyone's needs in the prayer section of their notebooks. Then pray aloud about these needs as members pray silently.

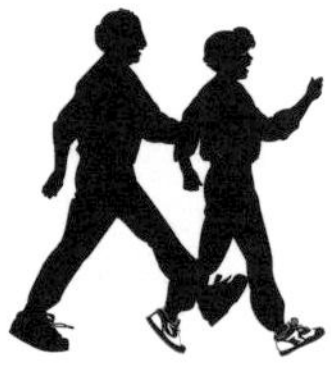

Session 6:

Certainly I'm Not Ever Dishonest . . . Am I?

GUIDING PRINCIPLE: I can change if I'm honest about my dishonesty.

Dear Leader:
Most of us consider ourselves to be very honest people. The purpose of this lesson is to point out some of the types of dishonesty so that we can inventory this condition in our lives. Even slight "slips" in honesty hinder our program of recovery. I have tried to focus on types of dishonesty that may be a problem for typical group members.

OPENING THE SESSION

OPENING PRAYER

Open with a brief prayer asking God to help members begin to think about their dishonesty.

APPLICATION QUESTION

Go around the circle letting members tell about the most important thing in their lives that is being crowded out by urgent things. So that there will be thought-provoking variety in the answers, tell members not to repeat an answer previously given, if possible.

PRINCIPLES FROM THE WORD

Here is my meditation for this week. It is on Proverbs 9:13-18, "The woman Folly is loud; she is undisciplined and without knowledge. She sits at the door of her house, on a seat at the highest point of the city, calling out to those who pass by, who go straight on their way. 'Let all who are simple come in here!' she says to those who pass by, who go straight on their way. 'Let all who are simple come in here!' she says to those who lack judgment. 'Stolen water is sweet; food eaten in secret is delicious!' But little do they know that the dead are there, that her guests are in the depths of the grave."

I identify with Folly. She is . . .

- *loud*
- *undisciplined*
- *without knowledge*
- *a show-off*
- *diverting others from their goals*
- *asking others to join her in her futile deeds*
- *telling lies about food*
- *enticing others to binge with her*

I used to be like that. I wasted my time running my mouth (though having little useful to say), being a bad influence, encouraging others to binge with me.

Father, thank you that you have given me purpose and are changing me from one like Folly to the woman you are calling me to be. She is . . .

- *one with a gentle and quiet spirit*
- *disciplined*
- *knowledgeable*
- *pointing to you, not self*
- *encouraging others to establish goals and to use their time wisely*
- *asking others to join you*
- *telling them the truth about food . . . that food eaten in secret is damaging, and healthy eating brings life.*

Lord, I do praise you for directing me along right paths and turning me from spending my days in folly.

STEPPING FORWARD

STEPPING STONE SURVEY

This week's focus is on Journaling and how it helps us spend our time, calories, and money more efficiently. Lead the discussion on this topic, using the information provided below.

- Have your Time Management List (see last week) handy to show the class and ask if anyone else has done his or hers. Don't explain how to do it in class, but offer to help after class if someone would like to do it.
- A Victory List (refer members to Unit 2) is helpful because it reminds us of certain things that we want to remember to do daily. Have extra forms available.
- Journaling our food during the day (or the next morning) helps us spend our calories more efficiently. Also, planning ahead what we are going to eat is very helpful.
- Keeping an account of our activities each day takes about 30 seconds, but is helpful to see where our time is spent. We jot down on our Activity List (refer members to the back of their workbooks) anything significant that we do each day. We keep this in the section with our Time Management List.
- I have a stated goal for each day—just one important thing that I want to get done that day. I write it on my Victory List and tell my accountability partner what my goal is and if I did it.
- I also have a Money Management Sheet. Do you ever wonder where all your money goes? Our Step Forward Money Management Sheet is included in the handouts (refer members to the back of their workbooks). It takes a few seconds every day to record these expenditures and helps me to stick to my budget. To use the Money Management Sheet—every morning do the following:

1. Record the amount of cash you have on hand.
2. Record any money you received (for example, checks cashed).
3. Record the money spent under the appropriate column. There is a space to write in family members' names on the right.

SPIRITUAL FOCUS

We will continue our Fourth Step inventory by discussing dishonesty, taking a close look at four types: stealing, cheating, breaking laws, and lying.

Stealing

What are some examples of stealing?
- Theft—of things, ideas, or work
- Shoplifting
- Income taxes
- Expense account
- Not working while being paid to work
- Taking supplies from the office
- Taking advantage of another's mistake (for example, being given too much change)
- Taking advantage of another's ignorance (There is a fine line between making an honest profit and taking advantage of another. Only the Holy Spirit can guide you in distinguishing between the two.)

Cheating

What are some examples of cheating?
- On tests
- On a food plan
- On a commitment

Type of Commitment	How One Cheats on That Commitment
• Marriage	*Emotional or physical adultery, slandering spouse*
• Contract	*Not paying bills and so forth*
• Verbal Commitment	*Not keeping your word to another*
• Commitment to God	*After repentance, continue the sin*

Breaking Laws

What type of laws do Christians tend to break most often?
Traffic laws.

Lying

Who do we lie to?
- To ourselves
- To another
- To God

Types of lies: Can you think of an example for each one?
- **Bold lies:** We all know what bold lies are.
- **White lies:** lies that "don't hurt anyone." Of course, we know that all lies are sin and they do hurt someone, usually ourselves.
- **Half-truths:** omitting the truth when not asked (not mentioning a mistake or sin), exaggerating, minimizing.
- **Rationalization:** providing a plausible but untrue reason for your conduct.
- **Denial:** lying about a problem to yourself.
- **Slander:** making untrue statements about someone.
- **Pretending:** mask-wearing (not letting people know you); hypocrisy (pretending to be one way while being another; flattery (false or exaggerated compliments). "Acting as if" is claiming one of God's promises, not pretending.

What are some causes of lies?
- Bad habit
- Fear of punishment
- Fear of rejection
- To control (wanting our own way)
- Wanting the easy way
- People pleasing, to keep peace
- Not wanting to hurt feelings
- To get revenge
- To protect—from embarrassment and shame
- To be more interesting, to impress

List the ways we tend to be dishonest in program:
- Lying about what we eat, omitting slips, binges
- Blaming our poor program on someone else
- Rationalizing or excusing our overeating
- Appearing to work a good program when we're not
- Not telling someone when they hurt our feelings

What are the results of dishonesty?
Group members will find the answers in the Bible verses in this section. **Have them take turns reading a verse and telling what result of dishonesty is found in that verse.**

Titus 1:11—You are a bad influence on others.

Luke 16:10—The sin of dishonesty grows.

1 Timothy 4:2—Your conscience is dulled, and you tend to sin more.

1 Timothy 6:10—You wander away from God, and this causes many griefs when you are dishonest in financial dealings.

Proverbs 28:10—You become a victim of your own dishonesty.

Proverbs 11:1—God does not delight in you when you are dishonest.

Ephesians 4:25a, 27, 28a—The devil gets a foothold.

Psalm 62:4b–5—Dishonesty takes away our peace.

1 Peter 3:10–11—We don't love life and will experience decreased serenity.

1 Peter 3:12—God turns his face from us and won't hear our prayers if we are in willful, unconfessed sin.

Apply Steps 1–5 to turning away from dishonesty.

Step 1: I'm powerless over my tendency to be dishonest, and it makes my life unmanageable.

Step 2: God can forgive me and help me to turn from it.

Step 3: I surrender my dishonesty to him and trust in his forgiveness and ability to help me to be honest.

Step 4: I will make a thorough inventory of it this week.

Step 5: I will confess it to God and another.

PHYSICAL FOCUS

Go around the circle letting members talk about how dishonesty has affected their weight.

CLOSING THE SESSION

STEPS FORWARD

As time permits, encourage anyone who is eating better or who has lost weight to tell about his or her *step forward.*

PRACTICING THE PRINCIPLES

Point out to members the homework assignments under "Practicing the Principles" in their workbooks. **Encourage members to work the assignments before the next meeting.**

PRAYER REQUESTS

Ask the members if anyone has specific needs that he or she would like lifted in prayer this week. Remind group members to make a note of everyone's needs in the prayer section of their notebooks. Then pray aloud about these needs as members pray silently.

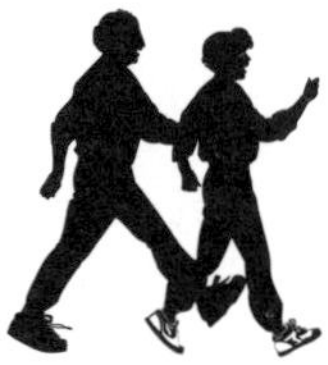

Session 7:

I'm Scared!

GUIDING PRINCIPLE: I can turn from fear if I revere the Lord.

Dear Leader:
One of the most important things that we can share with those in our group is the importance of fearing the Lord, not in a legalistic way of working hard to deserve his favor, but by remembering who he is and by putting his will for us first in our lives. We are taking inventory of two separate things this week: how much we fear the Lord and how much we fear our circumstances. Be on guard that as we focus on our fears, we don't become overwhelmed and forget God's provision. This will give Satan a foothold and can disrupt the class. Did you know that there are 365 "fear not!" verses in the Bible? I'll bet God knew that we would need one for every day of the year.

OPENING THE SESSION

OPENING PRAYER

Open with a brief prayer asking God to help members begin to see that by revering the Lord, they can turn from fear.

APPLICATION QUESTION

I really debated about the topic this week. I thought it might be too threatening to ask members to share current dishonesty with the group. It will be very important for them to do this with the recipient of their Fifth Step later, however.

PRINCIPLES FROM THE WORD

My meditation this week is from Micah 6:10-14, "Am I still to forget, O wicked house, your ill-gotten treasures and the short ephah, which is accursed? Shall I acquit a man with dishonest scales, with a bag of false weights? Her rich men are violent; her people are liars and their tongues speak deceitfully. Therefore I have begun to destroy you, to ruin you because of your sins. You will eat but not be satisfied; your stomach will still be empty. You will store up but save nothing, because what you save I will give to the sword."

Father, help me to confess and turn from any dishonesty in my life because I fear your wrath. Sometimes I get so carried away with the concept of your grace and mercy that I make you into a one-sided God. I pretend that you are some easy-to-fool grandfather who either doesn't notice my sins or ignores them. You do neither! When I am living in unconfessed sin, I often experience your displeasure in my empty stomach—I eat and am not satisfied. When I am in that state and the obsession with food begins, help me to stop and inventory the preceding hours and days for dishonesty and other sins in which I may be walking.

I thank you so much that the remedy is simple—confession and repentance. It is simple but not easy. It hurts me, after all these years, to see that I still fall so easily into sin. God, help me to walk in right relationship with you, without the walls that my dishonesty builds between us.

STEPPING FORWARD

STEPPING STONE SURVEY

This is a good time to encourage members to keep coming back. It is better to *step forward* a little than to fall backwards, so auditing is better than quitting.

How does someone audit Step Forward?

Julie says: *"I can audit Step Forward like a college class that I want to take, but don't want to take the tests or do the homework. I can show up for the class and listen, but not spend any time at home studying and doing the assignments. I learn a lot, but not as much as I would if I took the class in the regular way. It is much better to audit Step Forward (come to the meetings without doing homework or working the program) than it is not to come. I have seen many members who, after auditing Step Forward, have started working program. Even though it took awhile to get started, many of them lose weight and have wonderfully changed lives.*

How are you stepping forward?

Ask members to write yes or no next to each question as you read it out loud. Then have them follow the instructions after the quiz to evaluate where they are *stepping forward* the most, and where they are *stepping forward* the least.

How do you know if you are "passing" the course?

You are passing if you are getting better and *stepping forward* in any way.

- Take the quiz in the workbook. See if you are improving in all three areas.
- Ask yourself how you are doing on your Lab Courses.
- Pray and ask God how he thinks you are doing. (Note: It is important that the impatient and perfectionists do not let themselves get frustrated and overwhelmed because they are not seeing immediate results in all areas or because they are not doing it all perfectly.)

Do you grade yourself on a curve?

No. That requires comparing your progress with other members.

Have members recall from memory the nine Stepping Stones.

Journaling, Honesty, Confidentiality, Prayer, Reaching Out, Fellowship, Accountability, Scripture, and Food Plan.

SPIRITUAL FOCUS

We will finish our Fourth Step inventory by discussing fear.

Explain this statement: "Fear God, but don't be afraid!"

We are commanded repeatedly in the Bible to fear the Lord. It is important to understand what that means—to revere him, to be in awe of him, to worship and praise him. We are also commanded not to be afraid—not to fear our circumstances, our weaknesses, or our feelings.

Explain this statement: "Fear God, and you have nothing else to fear."

If one truly fears God in the right way, not with aversion or dread, but with awe and reverence, then the fears of this world will diminish. What people think about you, what you have or don't have, what your circumstances are, will pale in comparison with the importance of having a personal relationship with the King and Creator of the entire universe! As you grow in trust and confidence in his sovereignty and his sufficiency, you will know that his promises are true, and all of your needs will be met, all of your pain will be purposeful and bearable, and you will be secure and satisfied.

How does one show that he or she really fears the Lord?

One begins to experience each of the following more: (This is a process—often it is a very slow one. As we learn to keep our eyes on the Lord and work program, these things happen if we don't give up.)

- Decreased dread, increased serenity
- Desire to spend time with God
- Obey his Word more
- Hunger for his Word
- Desire to praise and worship God throughout the day
- Rely on God more

What does the Bible promise those who fear the Lord?

Go around the circle and take turns reading these.

What are the other types of fear?

Go around the circle letting members read the list and its examples. Point out that fears may be for yourself or for a loved one.

Can you find the antidote to fear that is mentioned in the following Scripture?

Trusting God is the antidote to fear.

What things must we realize in order to trust God?

- As Christians, God loves us unconditionally. He forgives our sins when we confess them.
- God desires the very best for us.
- God is sovereign. There is nothing that he can't do!
- God has wonderful plans for us.
- God will enable us to do his will as we abide in him.

Apply Steps 1–5 to help overcome fear.

Step 1: I admit that I am powerless over situations that I fear. Fear makes my life unmanageable.

Step 2: I believe that God, through Jesus Christ, can restore that feeling of peace I so desire. He can take care of everything that I fear.

Step 3: I am making a decision to turn my fears and everything that I dread over to his care and trust him to take care of me.

Step 4: This week I will recognize my fears and stop to write an inventory of them.

Step 5: I will share this inventory with God and another person.

If time permits after the Physical Focus, **let the members take turns reading the Bible verses that can help us overcome our fears. Ask them to circle their favorites.** Point out that we are to choose five of these verses for our homework meditations.

PHYSICAL FOCUS

Go around the circle letting members talk about their fears of losing weight and God's truth concerning these fears. Provide the answers below as needed.

Fear of temptation: If I were thin, I may be tempted to do things that God does not want me to do.

> **Truth:** We know that God will help us with any temptation, just as he is helping us overcome our temptation to eat too much.

Fear of intimacy: If I were thin, I wouldn't have a protective coating to shield me. (This faulty thinking often seems true for people who have been sexually abused as children.)

Truth: We know that God has created us to be close to others. We isolate, wear masks, and hide in food. This is not what God wants for us; he wants us to be emotionally intimate and real with others. He does not want us to be physically intimate with anyone other than our spouse. Obesity doesn't solve this problem; it just creates bigger ones.

Fear of change: "At least now I know what life is like." For some who have been obese for a long time, fear of change is a very real issue.

Truth: We learn that as we confess these fears to the Lord and to our coach, step out in faith, and work our program one day at a time, the changes that come are a blessing.

Fear of feeling our feelings: We numb our feelings with food. We are distracted from our problems when we are eating. We experience companionship with our binge buddies. Life is great! Or is it?

Truth: When we face our feelings, while working our program we will not be overwhelmed by them. One day at a time, with God's help and the support of our Step Forward group, we can do it.

CLOSING THE SESSION

STEPS FORWARD

As time permits, encourage anyone who is eating better or who has lost weight to tell about his or her *step forward*.

PRACTICING THE PRINCIPLES

Call attention to the homework assignments under "Practicing the Principles."

PRAYER REQUESTS

Ask if members have specific needs that they would like lifted in prayer this week. Remind them to make a note of everyone's needs in the prayer section of their notebooks. Then pray aloud about these needs as members pray silently.

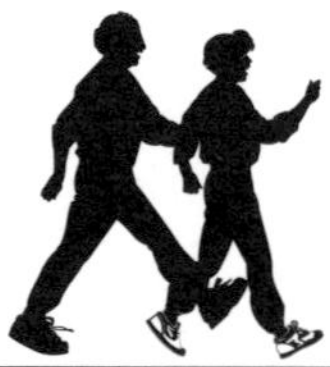

Session 8:

Summming It Up!

GUIDING PRINCIPLE: Step 5: I can get rid of things weighing me down if I do the Fifth Step.

Dear Leader:

It is important that as we prepare to summarize our Fourth Step and share it in the Fifth Step, we do so in the light of Steps 1, 2, and 3. It would be so easy for us to go back to our old shame-based legalism, trying to win God's favor. We already have his favor! We are his beloved children; therefore, we are free to look at our mistakes and our sins and confess them, praising God all the more for his wonderful provision for us on the cross. We gladly say, "I can't!" "God can!" "I'll let him!" What a relief when we look at our inventories that we don't have to change ourselves. We only have to rely on him and let him do the impossible in us. As we work the program, he'll keep giving us the desire and ability to do more and more of his will.

OPENING THE SESSION

OPENING PRAYER

Open with a brief prayer asking God to help members get rid of things weighing them down by doing their Fifth Step.

APPLICATION QUESTION

Go around the circle letting members tell what their worst fear is, how they are *stepping forward* away from it, and which Scripture helps them overcome it.

PRINCIPLES FROM THE WORD

My meditation is from Romans 8:15-16, "For you did not receive a spirit that makes you a slave again to fear, but you received the Spirit of sonship. And by him we cry, '*Abba*, Father.' The Spirit himself testifies with our spirit that we are God's children. Now if we are children, then we are heirs — heirs of God and co-heirs with Christ, if indeed we share in his sufferings in order that we may also share in his glory."

O God, I know who would love for me to be a slave again to fear! He sends his spirit to counteract the hope and power of your Holy Spirit, but I can stand firm against it by focusing on you.

Abba—Daddy, as I climb into your lap and hug your neck, I feel safe and secure from all of my fears. I know that if I have a problem, you will help me with it. If I fail, you will fix things so that they will be right. If I don't know what to do, you will whisper the right answer in my ear.

I know that my life won't be a failure, though I will often make mistakes, because I am your child. I can come to you, and you'll hold me and love me and set me back on the right path when I fail. You won't ridicule me or reject me, but continue to encourage me and stand by me.

STEPPING FORWARD

STEPPING STONE SURVEY

Go around the circle and ask members to share the question that shows the area of their greatest recovery.

SPIRITUAL FOCUS

This session we will summarize the Fourth Step and prepare to take Step 5.

What is the Fourth Step?

Made a searching and fearless moral inventory of ourselves.

What must you keep in mind while you are doing it?

The first three steps.
- I can't change my character defects.
- God can change them.
- I'll let him as I work my program of recovery and learn to surrender them to him.

What keeps you from doing a good fourth step?

Let the members take turns reading these.

Where do you begin a Fourth Step?

Look back at significant circumstances of your past. We have had the opportunity to write about our past in Unit 1, Week 1, and in Unit 2, Weeks 7, 8, and 9.

Encourage members to briefly describe (in writing) their childhood and their lives before Step Forward sometime this week, if they did not do so earlier.

Inventory the present by examining the following character defects:

Point out the list of character defects. Remind members that if they are struggling with a particular character defect, it might be helpful to refer back to the session when it was covered.

Preparing to Share Your Fourth Step

Read over this material in class. Use this time to encourage everyone to do a Fourth and Fifth Step and to use the next week or two to prepare.

Taking or Receiving the Fifth Step

What is promised in the Bible when one does the Fifth Step?

Go around the circle taking turns reading the Scriptures and answering the question.

- ***Proverbs 28:13***—Mercy (from God and sometimes from another)
- ***James 5:16***—Healing (spiritual, emotional, and physical); our prayers are effective
- ***Hebrews 10:22–25b***—Cleansing from a guilty conscience, being purified by God, and encouraging each other
- ***Luke 15:18b–19a***—Reconciliation
- ***Acts 19:18, 20***—The Word spreads and grows in power

Fifth Step Instructions

Read these in class.

PHYSICAL FOCUS

Go over aversion therapy in class. **Encourage the group members to practice it this week.**

CLOSING THE SESSION

STEPS FORWARD

Invite any members who are seeing progress in *stepping forward* to share their experiences with the group.

PRACTICING THE PRINCIPLES

Call attention to the homework assignments under "Practicing the Principles."

PRAYER REQUESTS

Ask if members have specific needs that they would like lifted in prayer this week. Remind them to make a note of everyone's needs in the prayer section of their notebooks. Then pray aloud about these needs as members pray silently.

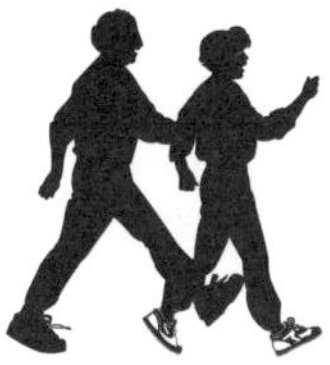

Session 9:

Why Do I Keep Doing Such Dumb Things?

GUIDING PRINCIPLE: Step 6: I can become ready to change if I look at what I'm doing to myself.

Dear Leader:

What a thought! We won't be ready to change unless we realize that our defects are harming us more than they are "helping" us. When we continue to live in denial of what our sin is doing to us, we will live in vicious cycles permanently. The barriers between us and God will remain. Let's do Sixth Step work this week to keep that from happening!

OPENING THE SESSION

OPENING PRAYER

Open with a brief prayer asking God to help members begin to look at what they are doing to themselves so that they can become ready to change.

APPLICATION QUESTION

Go around the circle letting members talk about their character defects. Encourage members to share a few positive steps they plan to take to overcome this defect.

PRINCIPLES FROM THE WORD

The meditation that I chose this week was Psalm 32:1–5, "Blessed is he whose transgressions are forgiven, whose sins are covered. Blessed is the man whose sin the Lord does not count against him and in whose spirit is no deceit. When I kept silent my bones wasted away through my groaning all day long. For day and night your hand was heavy upon me; my strength was sapped as in the heat of summer. Then I acknowledged my sin to you and did not cover up my iniquity. I said, 'I will confess my transgressions to the Lord'—and you forgave the guilt of my sin."

Lord, how blessed I am that you forgive all of my sins, that Jesus' perfect atonement covers them and you don't count them against me.

Help me to not be deceitful. As I do my Fourth and Fifth Steps, help me to be honest about all of my sins. My bones don't waste away as quickly as my commitment to healthy living when I am not honest with you.

I remember the days before I began my program of recovery when I used to groan all day long. I was so deep in denial, I didn't even know I had unconfessed sin in my heart. Through my program you have taught me how to come out of denial and to recognize my sin so I can confess it. But sometimes, Lord, I still go back to my old ways. Sin has such an insidious way about it. It sneaks up on me, and I don't know that it's there until I feel tormented again. My strength is sapped, and I feel weighted down, not knowing if it's your hand or Satan's that is upon me.

Help me to recognize all of my sins and confess them freely to myself, to you, and to my accountability partner as I take my Fifth Step.

STEPPING FORWARD

STEPPING STONE SURVEY

Encourage members to recite the Stepping Stones without looking at their notes. After each one is mentioned, let them relate it to the Fourth and Fifth Steps. Provide the answers below as needed.

- **Journaling.** I must use this Stepping Stone as I do my Fourth Step because I write my inventory.
- **Honesty.** Without this Stepping Stone, my Fourth and Fifth Steps are a waste of time. When I use honesty as I share, I will experience many blessings and will be able to continue on the rest of my journey one step at a time.
- **Confidentiality.** I know that what I say to someone in program will go no further because of this Stepping Stone. Therefore, I can share my character defects without fear.
- **Prayer.** I must bathe my Fourth and Fifth Steps in prayer so that I will not become overwhelmed as I look at my character defects.
- **Reaching Out.** When I get together with someone in program to do my Fifth Step, I am reaching out. It is possible to do this on the phone, but better to do it in person.
- **Food Plan.** If I refrain from compulsive overeating as I prepare to do my Fourth and Fifth Steps, I will be able to think more clearly.
- **Accountability.** I may choose to do my Fifth Step with my accountability partner or coach. The trusting relationship that we have established helps me to be honest.
- **Scripture.** God's Word guides me and lets me know when I am doing things that I need to confess.
- **Fellowship.** In my meetings I learn how to do my Fourth and Fifth Steps, and I am encouraged to do them.

SPIRITUAL FOCUS

This week we will begin the Sixth Step: Were entirely ready to have God remove all these defects of character.

Why is it hard to be "entirely ready" to have God remove all of our defects?

- Many of our defects are enjoyable.
- We won't fit in with others if we give them up.
- We don't think we can change.
- We might be ridiculed by old "friends" if we change.
- It is easier to do things like we always have.
- We fear living without them. We don't know what it would be like.

How Can We Make Ourselves Entirely Ready?

Decide if we really want to be healed of these defects.
Have a volunteer read this Scripture. Lead the discussion on the questions that follow.

What excuses did the invalid make?
- "No one will help me."
- "People get ahead of me."

What excuses do you make about continuing to compulsively overeat?
- "I can't help myself."
- "I don't overeat. I just have a slow metabolism."
- "My mother and aunts were all compulsive overeaters."
- "My life is just too hard right now to diet."

What is Jesus saying to us in these verses?
His exact words: "Get up! Pick up your mat and walk."

What he means: "There's no way you can do it unless you try. When I am here, you can do things you never dreamed that you'd be able to do!"

We examine each character defect to help us decide if we are entirely ready to have God remove our defects. What two questions do we need to ask about each defect?

1. How does each one "help" us? (Often we live the lie that it really does help us in some way.)
2. How does each one harm us?

When will we begin to be ready to let God remove each defect?
We will be ready to let God remove each defect only when we realize that it is doing more harm than good.

Have group members look at the list of character defects. Go through a few of these defects with the group until they get the idea. Don't try to do the whole list in class. I am not trying to include all of the answers here. I am just giving an example of each. Members will be asked to do a more complete list for homework of what some of their defects are doing to "help" them and to harm them. Reinforce the idea that the defects are not really helping us, but since we keep doing them, we are acting like they are.

We must be willing to change. What are some obstacles to change?

- Not stopping to realize why our lives are so unmanageable.
- Not willing to change because of fear of the unknown.
- Thinking that God won't (can't) change us.
- Wanting our own way.
- Not knowing how to change. Trying to change with willpower.
- Fear of losing control of our lives.
- Afraid others won't like us.
- Wanting a quick, painless remedy.

PHYSICAL FOCUS

Go around the circle with these three questions if you have time. If your time is limited, you may choose to ask only the first question.

CLOSING THE SESSION

STEPS FORWARD

Ask for volunteers to say encouraging things about how their program is helping them. Remind members that our aim is not to do everything perfectly. It is to *step forward* a little every day.

PRACTICING THE PRINCIPLES

Call attention to the homework assignments under "Practicing the Principles."

PRAYER REQUESTS

Ask if members have specific needs that they would like lifted in prayer this week. Remind them to make a note of everyone's needs in the prayer section of their notebooks. Then pray aloud about these needs as members pray silently.

Session 10:

Why Should I Change?

GUIDING PRINCIPLE: I can understand my defects if I study my temperament.

Dear Leader:

How many times do we think that we're completely ready to surrender something to God and then grab it back at the last minute? This precious little poem describes an incomplete Sixth Step beautifully! The author is unknown.

As children bring their broken toys,
With tears for us to mend,
I brought my broken dreams to God,
Because he was my friend.
But then, instead of leaving him,
In peace to work alone,
I hung around and tried to help
With ways that were my own.
At last, I snatched them back and cried,
"How can you be so slow?"
"My child," he said,
"What could I do? You never did let go."

Let's try to remember that the focus of the Sixth Step is on God, as he is the one who is going to remove our shortcomings. Our job is to be ready to let him do it!

OPENING THE SESSION

OPENING PRAYER

Open with a brief prayer asking God to help members begin to understand their defects by studying their temperaments.

APPLICATION QUESTION

In case there are people who didn't attend last week, explain the concept of how a defect can "help" you and harm you before asking these questions. **Then go around the circle letting members take turns talking about which character defects affect them the most.** Be sure that the second part of the question is also answered.

PRINCIPLES FROM THE WORD

Here is my meditation for this week. It is on John 15:1–2, 5, "[Jesus said,] 'I am the true vine, and my father is the gardener. He cuts off every branch in me that bears no fruit, while every branch that does bear fruit, he prunes so that it will be even more fruitful. . . . I am the vine; you are the branches. If a man remains in me and I in him, he will bear much fruit; apart from me you can do nothing.'"

Lord, I think of my mums when I read this passage. Nancy told me to pinch them back when the tiny blossoms begin to form because they will bush out and produce so much more. I did that, and I enjoyed the results for months. Flowers were everywhere on beautiful well-shaped plants.

I hadn't noticed a mum down the hill, and I forgot to prune it. It is blooming now, but the skinny stalks can't hold their own weight, and the flowers are falling in the dirt. Lopsided and spindly, the plant looks divided and unbalanced.

Help me, Lord, to desire to be pruned by you as you cut back the unnecessary overgrowth in my life. Help me not to dread your pruning because I know that I will be more fruitful as a result of it. Help me to remain in you constantly. Apart from you I wither and die inside. Help me to be entirely ready for you to remove all my defects of character.

STEPPING FORWARD

STEPPING STONE SURVEY

How do the Stepping Stones help you to have the willingness to change that you need to complete the Sixth Step?

Lead a discussion on this topic. Provide the answers below as needed.

- **Journaling**—When I write Victory Lists and Action Plans, I can break the necessary changes down to small achievable baby steps.

- **Honesty**—Until I am honest about my defects and the harm that they are doing to me, I will never change.

- **Confidentiality**—Because I know that I will not be gossiped about, I feel free to take off my mask and admit what needs changing.

- **Prayer**—When I pray for willingness, God gives it to me.

- **Reaching Out**—When I reach out to encourage others, I am encouraged too. I am often inspired by them to try new things.

- **Food Plan**—When I eat right, I tend to think right. When I eat compulsively, I continue in vicious cycles and ineffective behaviors.

- **Accountability**—When my partner asks me how I'm doing with my defects, I am encouraged to let go of them and to let God change them.

- **Scripture**—The promises help me to know what wonderful things will happen when I change.

- **Fellowship**—In my group I am encouraged to change when I see *steps forward* that others are making or I hear about the pain that their defects are causing them.

SPIRITUAL FOCUS

This session we will begin to look at the Sixth Step.

Let volunteers read the three things that we must do to make ourselves ready to change.

Tell the group: "Often, we are not ready to change because defects are fun, easy, and familiar. We don't understand that God will help us every step of the way. We are afraid of change, deprivation, and pain and don't understand that when we're doing things his way, we find joy and peace we've never known."

Decide what promises found in each of the following verses motivate us to change.

Go around the circle taking turns reading the Scriptures and, after each verse, ask the group what promise motivates us to change.

1 Peter 2:1–2—I will mature in my walk with the Lord.

Galatians 5:1—I will have freedom from slavery.

1 John 5:3-4a—I will show God that I love him.

Matthew 5:16—I will be a good witness.

Deuteronomy 30:15–16—I will choose not to be destroyed by sin. God will bless me.

Deuteronomy 30: 19b–20c—I will really live! My kids will too. I won't have barriers between me and God so that I will be able to love him more, hear his voice, and feel close to him.

What are some ineffective motivations for change?

- To manipulate God. ("I've been good to you, so you have to do this or that for me.")
- To impress others by my purity. (pride)
- To earn God's love. (legalism)
- To be able to love myself. (shame)

Temperaments: Let the group members take turns reading these (from *Personality Plus,* by Florence Littauer, Fleming H. Revell, a division of Baker Book House Company, Grand Rapids, Michigan).

Why is it so helpful to understand temperaments?

- I can quit beating myself up because of my natural tendencies.
- I can understand my strengths and weaknesses better.
- I can understand why others do the things they do and be more tolerant of them.

Why is temperament a Sixth Step issue?

I can understand why some defects are harder for me to let go of.

How can my positive traits produce negative results?

The answers follow:
1: b   2: a   3: d   4: c

PHYSICAL FOCUS

In order to review doing Action Plans, do a sample Action Plan together concerning compulsive overeating. See example on page 50 in this leader's guide. Remind members that the problem must be your own problem, and the goal must be realistic and as measurable as possible. Ask members to write actions they are willing to try.

Review how we do the Victory List by using the form included with the handouts in the **Unit 2 Leader's Guide**. List specific actions you want to do daily. Remind members not to make their goals too difficult and not to aim to do Victory Lists perfectly. The following are only a few suggestions for Victory List items as they relate to compulsive overeating. (We often include other areas on our Victory Lists, such as memorizing Scripture, writing letters, cleaning, and so forth.)

No sugar.
Twenty-five grams of fat.
No second helpings.
Wrote down what I ate.
Called my coach.

CLOSING THE SESSION

STEPS FORWARD

Ask for volunteers to say encouraging things about how their program is helping them. Remind members that our aim is not to do everything perfectly. It is to *step forward* a little every day.

PRACTICING THE PRINCIPLES

Point out the homework assignments under "Practicing the Principles" in their workbooks. **Encourage members to work the assignments before the next meeting.**

PRAYER REQUESTS

Ask the members if anyone has specific needs that he or she would like lifted in prayer this week. Remind group members to make a note of everyone's needs in the prayer section of their notebooks. Then pray aloud about these needs as members pray silently.

Action Plan

Problem	Goal	Actions
Compulsive overeating	Healthy eating by working program one day at a time!	1. Commit to a healthy food plan. 2. Write planned food daily. 3. Write actual food eaten daily. 4. Call coach one or more times a week. 5. Go to Step Forward weekly. 6. Make a Step Forward call daily. 7. 15 to 30 minutes quiet time daily. 8. 10-minute Bible assignment daily. 9. Half hour a week on Step Forward assignment. 10. Exercise 30 minutes three times a week. 11. Weigh once a week. 12. Memorize Scripture pertaining to Steps three minutes a day. 13. Be honest with myself and coach. 14. Pray for help in eating before each meal and when tempted. 15. No eating in front of TV. 16. When tempted: A. Ask myself, "Why do I feel empty?" Write! B. Make five-minute contracts with myself. C. Get out of the kitchen! D. Pray for willingness. E. Make a Step Forward call. 17. Have no binge foods in my house.

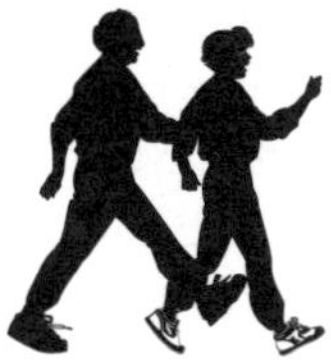

Session 11:

Boy, Do I Feel Humiliated!

GUIDING PRINCIPLE: Step 7: I can quit being humiliated if I understand humility.

Dear Leader:

This week we are starting the Seventh Step. We are asking God to remove our shortcomings. In our partnership we can't just ask him to do all the work and sit back and wait; there are many things that the Bible encourages us to do in order to be open to the changes that God is making in us. We don't want to live like a prisoner when the cell door has been unlocked. There is no way to know that the changes are occurring if we continue to act and talk as we always have. Often our feelings must follow our actions. That is why in our program of recovery, we are encouraged to "act as if." This is not encouraging hypocrisy, but it tells us to step out in faith and reliance on the Lord in the direction that he leads us, away from our shortcomings and toward the new way of life that he has prepared for us.

OPENING THE SESSION

OPENING PRAYER

Open with a brief prayer asking God to help members begin to understand humility so that they can quit being humiliated.

APPLICATION QUESTION

Go around the circle letting members share their dominant temperament and how it affects their character defects. Encourage members to keep their answers brief.

PRINCIPLES FROM THE WORD

Ask members to share their Scripture meditation. Here is my meditation for this week and my Sixth Step Prayer. It is from Romans 8:28–31, "And we know that in all things God works for the good of those who love him, who have been called according to his purpose. For those God foreknew, he also predestined to be conformed to the likeness of his son, that he might be the firstborn among many brothers. And those he predestined, he also called; those he called, he also justified; those he justified, he also glorified. What, then, shall we say in response to this? If God is for us, who can be against us?

> *You knew me before I was conceived. You have had a wonderful purpose planned for my life since before the earth was formed: that I would become more like Jesus. You have been wooing me to yourself since I took my first breath, and when Jesus was nailed to the cross, my sins were nailed there too—covered and forgiven. Since the beginning of time you have been preparing for my homecoming, for you knew that I would someday go to heaven to be with you. Time means nothing to you; a thousand yesterdays are as a day.*
>
> *As I think of your eternal plan for my life, I can rest assured. Taking my Sixth Step—being entirely ready to have you remove my defects and put Jesus' qualities in their place—is the only natural and right thing to do. All of the days of my life have come to a culmination at*

this life-changing step:

I am ready to turn.

I am ready to change.

I am ready to grow.

I am entirely ready to have you remove all of my defects of character. You are for me, Lord. Nothing I have done, nothing I will do, no one I have known or will know can change your purpose for my life.

STEPPING FORWARD

STEPPING STONE SURVEY

How might each temperament type work his or her Step Forward program in an ineffective manner?

- A person with a **sanguine** temperament might talk too much at meetings, have problems with honesty because of wanting to please others and receive their approval; he or she might struggle with the discipline needed to work program. It would be especially important for that person to use a Victory List as a daily reminder of short-term goals and to have daily accountability.

- A person with a **choleric** temperament might want to take the lead in the discussions in group and with his or her coach. He or she might be unwilling to try new things, or might tend to use willpower and have problems admitting powerlessness. It would be helpful for him or her to have a coach who will be assertive in encouraging this person with a choleric temperament to try new things. It would also help the choleric to frequently practice saying, "I can't; God can; I'll let him."

- A person with a **melancholy** temperament might try to work program perfectly. He or she must be careful not to be a perfectionist when doing a Victory List. A melancholy person needs to watch that he or she doesn't get depressed over character defects.

- **A phlegmatic** person may tend not to share in meetings. He or she may have problems getting motivated to work program. It would be especially helpful to have a coach who is enthusiastic and encouraging.

SPIRITUAL FOCUS

This week we will look at the difference between humiliation and humility and how they relate to Step 7: Humbly asked him to remove our shortcomings.

Group members' workbooks have a list of some of the differences between humiliation and humility. Go over the first four of these in class.

Humiliation
Self worth based on what I do
Low self-esteem
Know-it-all, unteachable
False pride

Humility
Self worth based on whose I am
Contentment in what God is doing in me
Desiring to learn more
Pride in Christ in me

Point out the section in the workbook titled "What is humility?" Read this section out loud or have a volunteer read it out loud to the class.

What is my responsibility in this partnership?

Go around the circle letting the members read the Bible verses and discuss the accompanying questions. Provide the answers below as needed.

- **Philippians 4:6**

If God commands me not to worry, and I worry anyway, that just makes it worse because then I worry about worrying! What does he mean by these verses?
You are not at the mercy of your feelings. There are certain things you are encour-

aged to do when worried that will help you.

What specifically am I to do to turn from worry?
Offer prayers, petitions, give thanks, present requests to God.

What is the difference between prayer and petition?
Petition is often in writing, a more formal type of prayer.

How does this Scripture relate to the Seventh Step?
I am to pray and present my requests to God concerning my shortcomings with an attitude of thanksgiving that he will help me to turn from them.

- **Hebrews 12:11**

How does this relate to the Seventh Step?
As I am giving up old ways, I may go through a type of withdrawal. It won't be easy, but it will be worth it.

What do I have to keep in mind while I am learning new ways?
I have to be willing to go through the pain because the positive characteristics and serenity will be following.

- **Hebrews 12:12–13**

How does this relate to the Seventh Step?
I must work to establish good habits to replace bad ones. I must not make my recovery harder by placing stumbling blocks (a bag of cookies?) in my path. I need to use the Stepping Stones to make level paths for my feet.

What does "the lame may not be disabled" mean from a Seventh Step perspective?
Things can go from bad to worse if I don't take the Seventh Step by asking God to remove my shortcomings. They have already made me lame and will get worse if I don't do something.

- **2 Corinthians 10:5**

How does the first part of this verse relate to the Seventh Step?
I am not to argue against the instruction for my life that God gives me in the Bible or pretend by daydreaming and living in "if only's."

How does the second part of this verse relate to the Seventh Step?
When I am discouraged or feel hopeless, I'll recognize that these are not thoughts of recovery, and I'll capture the thoughts and turn them around to recovery thinking.

Am I becoming what God wants me to be? Am I running the Rat Race or the Right Race?
Ask volunteers to read these Scriptures that exhort us to *step forward*. Have group members read out loud these Scriptures and the comparisons between these two lifestyles.

How do I change races?
Read these to the group. On Steps 7–12, there is no need to discuss how each of the rest of the steps trains us to change into the Right Race, that of recovery. Just mention it.

PHYSICAL FOCUS

Love Hunger, by Drs. Minirth, Meier, Henfelt, and Sneed (Thomas Nelson, Nashville), talks about the roles that food plays.

What harm does it do when food becomes my . . .

- **Parent:** I am living a lie when I believe that food nurtures me like a parent. God takes care of all my needs and fills my hunger.

- **Idol:** When food is my idol, it comes between me and God because I cannot worship two things at the same time.

- **Best friend:** When I believe that food is my best friend, I am devastated when I finally realize that my best friend has betrayed me and is harming me.

- **Plaything:** When I think that food is a plaything, I am playing with fire. Food is not a toy. It can kill me.

- **Source of sensuality:** When it is my main source of sensuality, my other senses are ignored and dulled.

- **Mood-altering drug:** When I use it as a mood-altering drug, it numbs my pain, but because I am unable to think clearly, I am prevented from dealing with my pain constructively and I can't solve my problems.

CLOSING THE SESSION

STEPS FORWARD

As time permits, encourage anyone who is eating better or who has lost weight to tell about his or her *step forward.*

PRACTICING THE PRINCIPLES

Point out the homework assignments under "Practicing the Principles" in the workbooks. Encourage members to work the assignments before the next meeting.

PRAYER REQUESTS

Ask the members if anyone has specific needs that he or she would like lifted in prayer this week. Remind group members to make a note of everyone's needs in the prayer section of their notebooks. Then pray aloud about these needs as members pray silently.

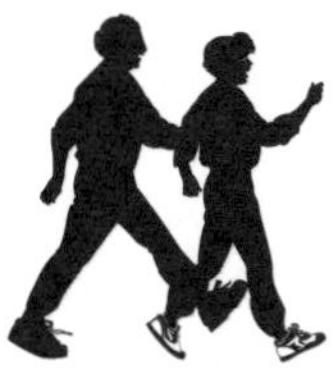

Session 12:

You Mean I'm Gifted?

GUIDING PRINCIPLE: I can use my gifts if I let God have my shortcomings.

Dear Leader:

As we take our Seventh Step, and God begins to remove our shortcomings, the spiritual gifts that have been in us since we accepted Christ have room to grow. Just as we don't have to remove our own shortcomings, but rely on God to do that for us, so we don't have to make our spiritual gifts materialize; that's God's job. We must trust him and rely on him as we begin to identify our gifts and learn how to use them.

OPENING THE SESSION

OPENING PRAYER

Open with a brief prayer asking God to help members let him have their shortcomings so that they can begin to use their gifts.

APPLICATION QUESTION

Go around the circle letting members talk about the implied command from the Scripture that encourages them most to let go and let God.

PRINCIPLES FROM THE WORD

My meditation this week is from Philippians 3:12 (Living Bible), "I don't mean to say I am perfect. I haven't learned all I should even yet, but I keep working toward that day when I will finally be all that Christ saved me for and wants me to be."

> *I forget sometimes. I don't have to be perfect. I can get so preoccupied, trying to do things right, my purpose changes, and my focus shifts to myself and my inability.*
>
> *Lord, I want to be the woman you want me to be. I really do want to keep working toward that day when I will finally be all you saved me for. Thank you for the Twelve Steps that teach me how to do that by growing in humble reliance on you.*
>
> *I know I'll never be able to say "I've arrived" until I get to heaven, but thanks to you, I am so much better than I was. I know there will always be struggles. I don't want to try to avoid them, but to continue to learn all you are teaching me through them.*
>
> *I want to continue to step forward toward you one day at a time. Help me to do that and to become all that you've called me for and want me to be.*

STEPPING FORWARD

STEPPING STONE SURVEY

Go around the circle letting members who want to talk about ways that they are *stepping forward*.

SPIRITUAL FOCUS

This session will discuss spiritual gifts: Don't be pulled into divisive denominational issues or try to answer all questions about spiritual gifts. Encourage everyone to think about gifts in light of what the Bible says and how God is leading each of them to use his or her gifts for God's glory. If we come from different denominations, we most likely will not agree on certain points. God wants unity in his church, not uniformity. To avoid controversy and because of limited time, we will not talk about all of the spiritual gifts, only those found in Romans 12:6-8. If members want to take a more complete gifts inventory, suggest that they ask their minister to give them one.

Why discuss spiritual gifts with the Seventh Step?

We discuss spiritual gifts with the Seventh Step because God is beginning to remove our shortcomings. Now there is room for his gifts that have been neglected (or smothered with peanut butter). As we become more aware of the gifts he has given us and we use them by relying on God, we will draw closer to him. When we are abiding in the Lord, we will not be drawn back into our old ways as easily.

Let volunteers read the two Bible verses. Lead a discussion on the questions that follow. Provide the answers below as needed.

Who has spiritual gifts?

All Christians have at least one spiritual gift.

What is their purpose?

Their purpose is to share the grace that God has given us with others and to build up the church.

What should their ultimate result be?

The ultimate result will be that God will be praised through Jesus Christ.

What is the difference between a talent and a spiritual gift?

A talent is a natural ability. A spiritual gift is an ability that God gives us that will build up the church and glorify God through Christ. For example, I may have a talent for teaching, but if I am not using it to teach others about Jesus, then it is not considered to be a spiritual gift.

Read Romans 12:6-8 out loud. **Ask members to underline the gifts mentioned before going on.** Briefly read over the descriptions of these spiritual gifts.

How must I use my gifts?

Use each one with love.

Now that I know what my primary spiritual gift is, what do I do?

- Ask yourself if you are using your gift and pray for willingness to do the work God has prepared for you. (Do your homework this week!)
- Research a need for your gift in your group and church.
- Pray for wisdom, assess your time availability, and then volunteer. ***Julie says:*** *"Sometimes we have to volunteer to do something that is not using our gift at first. When I joined a new church a few years ago, the only 'spiritual gift' I was able to use was my ability to type. After getting to know the minister better, he realized that I have the gift of teaching, and it wasn't long until I was teaching classes there."*

What do I need to watch out for as I use my gift?

- Not to be prideful of our gifts.
- Not to be envious of others' gifts.
- Not to do them in the flesh. (We can go overboard on each spiritual gift; for example, mercy turns to rescuing, leadership turns to bossing, prophecy turns to controlling. We all know someone who has the gift of hospitality and practically crams food down our throats, not wanting to take no for an answer.)

- Not to think that just because it's easy for us, it's easy for everyone.

- Not to be critical of someone because of his or her gift, (for example, "He gives so much of his money away that he won't have enough for his old age.")

- Not to concentrate so hard on our gifts that we forget about our fruit. (The fruit of the Spirit: love, joy, peace, patience, kindness, goodness, faithfulness gentleness, self-control.)

- Not prioritizing right. Using our gifts to the detriment of our families. When we have a spouse or children, we must remember to leave plenty of quality time for them. ***Julie says:*** *"I remember a time in my life when I didn't do this. I thought that I was doing the right thing to be at the church every spare minute to teach, and so forth. After all, wasn't I using the gift that God had given me? The Lord very definitely pointed out that my family should come first, and I learned another valuable lesson."*

- Falling into false guilt because we are not doing as much as someone else (for example, when we hear a missionary speak, feeling guilty because we're not going to Africa even though we have spouses and children who don't want to go).

How can I understand my gifts from a Seventh Step perspective?

Let a volunteer read these in class.

PHYSICAL FOCUS

Following are the answers to the true or false test in the workbook. **Let the members check their answers during class.**

1. **False:** A Type C personality is at greater risk for cancer. This person is a people-pleaser who does not express anger.

2. **True:** With adequate support, signs of stress may be greatly diminished. This has been measured in clinical studies.

3. **True:** Under the advice of their physician, some who are chronically depressed might want to consider taking medication to elevate their serotonin level and going to a Christian counselor to help them deal with their depression. This may help their food cravings.

4. **False:** Chronic resentments can increase all of these. Resentments often decrease one's immune system, including immunity to infections.

5. **False:** Studies have shown that even having a pet to take care of can help people to live longer.

6. **True:** For example, a recent study of terminal breast cancer patients shows that those in support groups lived an average of 18 months longer than others.

7. **True:** When there is no disclosure and one doesn't share his or her true feelings, anxiety levels rise, and the ability to fight opportunistic infections diminishes.

8. **True:** Actors who were playing a happy role and later, a sad one, were studied. Their blood chemistry changed with each role, reflecting physiological stress of sadness, even though they were only acting.

9. **True.**

CLOSING THE SESSION

STEPS FORWARD

Invite any members who are seeing progress in *stepping forward* to share their experiences with the group.

PRACTICING THE PRINCIPLES

Point out to members the homework assignments under "Practicing the Principles" in their workbooks. Encourage members to work the assignments before the next meeting.

PRAYER REQUESTS

Ask the members if anyone has specific needs that he or she would like lifted in prayer this week. Remind group members to make a note of everyone's needs in the prayer section of their notebooks. Then pray aloud about these needs as members pray silently.

I hope you join us in the final unit and that you continue stepping forward with us!

Be sure to write to me and tell me about your progress.

My address:

Julie Morris
2663 Valleydale Rd.
Suite 266
Birmingham, AL 35244
email: stpforward@aol.com

MINI-GROUPS

*If some of your members are hesitant to get accountability partners, here's a wonderful addition to the meetings that will really help: **Mini-groups**.*

Read the following paragraphs and determine if you want to add this additional component to your meetings. Then give each mini-group leader the instructions found on the next page and the forms it mentions. (The forms can be found in the back of the Unit 2 Leader's Guide.)

At the end of each meeting, after you've finished your prayer time, divide into groups of three or four for 10-15 minutes. Assign a leader for each group. Lead one mini-group yourself. During each session, leaders and members will share with their mini-group how they stepped forward in the following areas:

- **Their eating**—If they have gotten off track during the week (not just slips, but bingeing or overeating daily), they will bring the mini-group leader an Off Track Form that they have filled out. If they have eaten according to their food plan consistently that week, the mini-group leader will give them an Award Sheet. Each member will save his or her Award Sheets in a certain part of his or her notebook. Each award sheet is worth a point. When members have collected 10 points, they may make a selection from the Gift Box.*
- **Their weight**—Members will report to their mini-group leader whether they have lost or gained weight that week. If they have lost weight, the mini-group leader will give them an Award Sheet stating the amount of weight they lost. Members are responsible to record their weight weekly on the dated weight page in their notebook, and mini-group leaders will record, for their records, how much weight the member has lost or gained each week. Members do not tell the mini-group leader how much they weigh, only whether they have lost or gained. Each pound lost from their original weight is worth one point toward a Gift Box selection. (Members will not receive points for losing weight they recently gained.)
- **Their commitment to step forward physically the next week** (for example, eliminating sugar that week, exercising a certain amount of time, or not eating in front of the TV). The mini-group leader will give an Award Sheet to members who have accomplished their commitment that week. Members may be rewarded up to three weeks for keeping the same commitment.
- **Their memory work assignment.** Every few weeks memory work will be a part of their homework assignment. Members will receive an Award Sheet if they are able to recite the memory work during the mini-group session.
- **Their forward stepping: Four Things That Help Stepping Forward** (being on time for the meeting, doing homework, sharing a meditation in class, and making a Step Forward call). Each week members will fill out *Forward Stepping Four*, the short form found with the handouts in your **Unit 2 Leader's Guide**. They will receive an Award Sheet if they accomplish these things.

  Members are never chastised if they do not do their assignments, accomplish their goals, or if they gain weight. **They are just encouraged** to step forward the following week.

** The purpose of the Gift Box is to reward members for stepping forward. Every month (or more often if needed) members will bring an inexpensive wrapped gift that will be placed in the Gift Box ($1-$2). Gift selections will be made during the main meeting before the prayer time so that everyone in the group may applaud their efforts.*

DEAR MINI-GROUP LEADERS,

During the first mini-group session:

- **Tell your members to weigh themselves each week.**

  Since mini-groups are just getting started, encourage them to weigh themselves the next day—before eating, without clothes, and record their weight and the date in their notebook. Although you're the leader of the mini-group, it is important for you to participate as well. Emphasize that you will not be telling each other your weight. You will only say how many pounds you've lost or gained that week. Ask them to be prepared during the next mini-group session to tell you the number of pounds they lost or gained during the week. If someone does not wish to participate in this part of the mini-group session, the person may pass.

- **Hand the members several Off Track Forms that your Step Forward leader will supply for you.**

  Suggest that they keep these in the food/weight section of their notebooks. Tell them to fill one out each time they get off track in their eating—not just slips, but bingeing or overeating daily. The Off Track Form is an excellent way to recognize negative patterns and overeating triggers, so encourage members to keep them to review from time to time.

- **Hand members a Commitment Form.**

  If they are willing to make a commitment to step forward physically the next week, ask them to share this commitment with the group and fill out the form. Some possible commitments might be eliminating sugar for the week, exercising a certain amount of time, or not eating in front of the TV. Suggest that they put the form in the prayer section of their notebook to remind them to pray each morning for the willingness and ability to do what they have committed to do that week. Next week and each week following, give an Award Sheet to members who have accomplished their commitment. It is best if they only make one commitment a week. Members may be rewarded up to three times for keeping the same commitment.

- **If there is a memory assignment the week you begin your mini-group (for example, verses, steps, information about fat grams and calories), ask if anyone would like to recite what he or she memorized.**

  If they are able to do it, give them an Award Sheet. Members will have the opportunity to recite new memory work during each mini-group session. They will not receive an Award Sheet for things they memorized before mini-groups were started.

- **Hand members a Forward Stepping Four form to see if they get an Award Sheet for accomplishing these four goals.**

  Give them an extra copy to put in their notebooks as a reminder so they can get an Award Sheet each week all four goals are reached.

As a mini-group leader, it is up to you to encourage your members to step forward. The best way to encourage others to step forward is by doing it yourself! It will also be very helpful if you call your members during the week and encourage them to call each other. Suggest they bring interesting articles about weight loss or other things that will help the group to work program.

Mini-group Leader Instructions

HOW TO COACH

If you were to ask a football coach how to coach, he would probably say, "I don't know how you are supposed to coach, but I know what works for me." We can take a clue from that statement. I can tell you what works for me, but you should coach as God leads you to. The only requirements are that you work the program yourself, don't pretend to do it perfectly, rely on God, and point to him.

Getting Started

Ask the person(s) you are coaching to call you once or twice a week at an appointed time. If any of your coachees is going through a hard time, however, you might touch base with that person every day for a while. Tell coachees that when they least want to call you is probably when they most need to do so.

When you agree to work together, make a list of things the coachee wants to be accountable for. She or he will likely report on some of the following:

- ***Food.*** If coachees are not ready to eat according to a food plan, don't try to make them do so. Find out what physical behaviors they are willing to be accountable for. For example, are they willing to remove from their house foods that trigger their binges?

- ***Quiet Time.*** Help coachees determine an achievable goal, but do not tell them what to do. If they have never had daily quiet time, fifteen minutes a day, five days a week is an acceptable goal.

- ***Homework Assignments.*** Your coachees may be accountable to spend fifteen to thirty minutes a week on homework assignments and to discuss them with you.

- ***Establishing Good Habits.*** Review the Stepping Stones with coachees and see what goals they would be accountable for to help them use the Stepping Stones. Be sure that the goals are achievable and that coachees don't set so many that they will be overwhelmed.

Some Do's and Don'ts

- **Do pray for guidance to know how much to listen and when to interrupt and focus on program.** You are responsible to point coachees to recovery. Don't encourage behavior such as gossip and self-pity by listening to too much of it.

- **Do realize that it is not your responsibility to fix what is wrong with your coachees.** You are simply to point out some right directions and to leave the rest up to God. Don't allow yourself to become overwhelmed by coachees' problems.

- **Do remind coachees frequently that they will not be able to work program perfectly.** Be watchful for perfectionist mindsets, which often are a stumbling block to working a good program. Also discourage legalism. Remind coachees that they work program to make a level path for their feet, not to win God's favor.

- **Don't be afraid to ask coachees for honest feedback** if they are upset over something you have said or if they are not willing to do an assignment or to try something that you have suggested.

- **Don't give advice.** If coachees bring a problem to you, encourage them to use the Stepping Stones and the Twelve Steps to work out a solution.

- **Do be a cheerleader, not a policeman.** Encourage coachees to make better choices, but don't criticize them.

Coaching Courtesy

As a rule coachees should call the coach, not the other way around.

Do not take a coachee's call about a problem when you are upset yourself. Say that you are not able to talk just then and that you will call back. If coachees call at any other time that is not a good time for you to talk, gently tell them so; but name a time when you will call them back.

Return all of coachees' calls. Each time you call them back, ask if this is a good time for them to talk.

Scenarios and Responses

- *Mary is angry with her husband and tells you, her coach, that she overeats because he wants her to lose weight.*
  Response: Encourage Mary to work through the Anger Action Plan from Session 6 Unit 1, and to study the Bible verses in that session to see what God would tell her about her situation.

- *Ellen wants to tell you about all the terrible things that are happening in her life. She wants to feel sorry for herself and doesn't want to talk about program.*
  Response: Try to focus on program. Before discussing circumstances, ask, "How have you used the Stepping Stones since we last talked?" Ask her to write about her situation. You may have to limit the amount of time that the two of you talk if she is deep into self-pity, since it is not good for her or for you to rehash difficult circumstances at length.

- *Susan, your new coachee, is upset because she binged last night.*
  Response: Ask Susan to write about the circumstances that led up to her binge. Ask that she then write what she learned from her mistake.

- *Bonnie gets upset with you every time you give her advice and refuses to do anything you suggest.*
  Response: You shouldn't be giving Bonnie advice. A better approach is to share your experiences in similar situations and to ask her to use the Stepping Stones and the steps. Ask what she is willing to do to work program.

When Coachees Flounder

When coachees are not doing well, ask:

- How have you been using the Stepping Stones?
- What did you learn from the mistake?
- Have you written this up in your journal?
- How are you willing to work program in this situation?

When coachees quit calling, pray and then call after a few days. After they have missed the second week, call again. Gently ask if they want to have a coach.

When coachees quit working program but still call, keep asking the above questions. Encourage them to pray for willingness to use the Stepping Stones. If they only want to dump their problems on you, tell them (after prayer) that you will coach them when they are ready to work program. Or tell them to call you when they have written an assignment you have given them concerning their problems (an Action Plan, prayer, Bible meditation, or the like).

Rewards of Coaching

Few things in life can bring more joy than coaching. It is exciting to watch as God changes your coachees and to feel that you have contributed to their transformation in some way.

STEP FORWARD!

YOU STEPPED FORWARD!

Awarded to

____

____

Date

For accomplishing the goals that you set for yourself with God's help for one week or for losing __________ pounds.

presented by

Julie Morris and

your Step Forward Group Leader

____

STEP FORWARD!

Tired of regaining lost pounds?

Learn how to get to the roots of your problem with food so that this time the extra pounds won't return.

STEP FORWARD
Christian Twelve Steps to Get Your Weight Off and *Keep It Off!*

Affordable nondenominational Bible study weight-loss program

Everyone is invited to the weekly classes.

Where:______________________________

When:______________________________

Cost:______________________________

Call for information:____________________